PENGUIN BOOKS

NO MORE MENSTRUAL CRAMPS
AND OTHER GOOD NEWS

Penny Wise Budoff, M.D., is in private practice on Long Island
and is Clinical Associate Professor of Family Medicine at the State
University of New York at Stony Brook. She lectures widely and
has frequently appeared on television to talk about new developments in women's health care. She has published research articles
in prominent medical journals. Dr. Budoff is married and has two
children.

No More Menstrual Cramps

and Other Good News

by

Penny Wise Budoff, M.D.

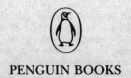

PENGUIN BOOKS

Penguin Books Ltd, Harmondsworth,
Middlesex, England
Penguin Books, 625 Madison Avenue,
New York, New York 10022, U.S.A.
Penguin Books Australia Ltd, Ringwood,
Victoria, Australia
Penguin Books Canada Limited, 2801 John Street,
Markham, Ontario, Canada L3R 1B4
Penguin Books (N.Z.) Ltd, 182–190 Wairau Road,
Auckland 10, New Zealand

First published in the United States of America by
G. P. Putnam's Sons 1980
First published in Canada by
Academic Press Canada Limited 1980
Published with revisions in Penguin Books 1981

LIBRARY OF CONGRESS CATALOGING IN PUBLICATION DATA
Budoff, Penny Wise.
No more menstrual cramps, and other good news.
Reprint. Originally published:
New York: Putnam, 1980.
Includes bibliographical references.
1. Gynecology—Popular works. I. Title.
[RG121.B89   1981]   618.1   81-2197
ISBN 0 14 00.5938 5   AACR2

Printed in tne United States of America by
Offset Paperback Mfrs., Inc., Dallas, Pennsylvania
Set in Video Baskerville

The author gratefully acknowledges permission from the following to reprint material in this book: *Behavior, Research, and Therapy,* for material from "The Development of the Menstrual Symptom Questionnaire," by M. D. Chesney and P. L. Tasto, Vol. 13; copyright © Pergamon Press, Ltd., 1975. The Carnation Company, Los Angeles, California, for the sodium-restricted diet plan. *International Journal of Gynecology & Obstetrics,* for a chart from "Life Risks Associated with Reversible Methods of Fertility Regulation," by Christopher Tietze and Sarah Lewit, 16:457; copyright © *International Journal of Gynaecology & Obstetrics,* 1979. *Journal of the American Medical Association,* for material from "Use of Mefenamic Acid in the Treatment of Primary Dysmenorrhea," by Penny W. Budotf, Vol. 241, No. 25 (June 22, 1979), pp. 2713–2716; copyright © American Medical Association, 1979.

Photograph #6 was taken by Rhoda Rosen; all other photographs were taken especially for this book by Anita F. Kirschner. The diagram on page 232 is by Joan Kasofsky.

Dedicated:

To all women
To our good health
To our success in achieving it
    By becoming medically informed
    By assuming an active responsibility for our bodies
    By pressuring for change as we see fit.

Contents

Illustration section follows page 158.

Acknowledgments

Writing a book is something like having a baby. It takes about the same length of time, and both are part of you. Because of this, my thank-yous for this newest addition will be in chronological order—as were the events and people who shaped my life.

That would mean that my first thanks go to my mother. Because of her sacrifices, I was able to go to medical school. Because of her ever-assured love, I was always secure. To her it was unimportant whether or not I was accomplished, I was loved simply because I was hers. I hope to convey that feeling to my own children so that they know its security. My love is their right and privilege, and does not have to be earned. I believe with this foundation, growth and ideals can best be achieved. Without that comforting knowledge, frustration and insecurity block life's real potential.

I want to thank the Ford Foundation Early Admissions Program. I won one of their four-year scholarships, which took me out of high school after my sophomore year and placed me in college. Because of the loss of my last two years in high school, I have some holes in my knowledge, but on the other hand, without the scholarship it is likely I never would have become a doctor.

Sy, my husband, comes next chronologically. He has been the single most important influence on my thinking. Because he had a working mother, my career was taken for granted. Indeed, he expected me to work. Sy is probably still more "lib" than I. This comes from his exquisitely keen sense of what is fair and right. His perception also helped me to better understand flaws in our system of medical care as he came to know them through his years of administering government health programs, and confirmed my ideas of unequal medical care based on sexual bias. Sy willingly pitched in and edited the first draft of this book into proper English as it came off my typewriter. He was an enormous help, as ever, both supportively and editorially.

I want to thank my children, Jeff and Cindy, for being such wonderful kids. They have never been awed by anything I have attempted—from being a pilot to writing a book. I am, to them, only their mother who loves them and takes care of their needs. First, I am expected to make sure that there is chocolate cake in the kitchen, and that help with piano practicing or social studies homework gets fitted into some time-slot or other. And so this book got written to a background of disco, and rock music, and piano practice. Life goes on, book manuscripts somehow get finished, but one job never ends—being a mother. My kids keep things in proper perspective. Because of them I am a better person—hassled maybe, but a better person.

Next, many thanks to Sheldon C. (Charlie) Sommers, M.D., who is a super pathologist and director of laboratories at Lenox Hill Hospital in New York City. I consider him a dear friend. We collaborated and published a paper on estrogen-replacement therapy in 1979. I have relied on his expertise and have drawn upon his material for my chapter on hysterectomy and "precancerous lesions."

Thanks to Hugh Barber, M.D., Chief of Obstetrics and Gynecology at New York Medical College, for his willingly given time and comments on my chapters on estrogen-replacement therapy and hysterectomy. I had qualms about submitting the chapter on hysterectomy to a gynecologist for proofreading because of the antisurgeon tone of the chapter. Dr. Barber wrote back, however, that my message was right on target and needed to be said.

Martin Stone, M.D., past president of the American Association of Obstetricians and Gynecologists, also immediately consented to proof two chapters for gynecologic correctness. He returned the chapters in person and said, "Kind of strong, aren't they? You're really sticking it to male gynecologists." Then he laughed and said, "Don't worry, the chapters are fine."

If two such prestigious gynecologists can agree that there is too much paternalism and too much unnecessary surgery, I can only hope that with continued exposure of the issues, change will come rapidly and women will have better care.

Dr. Leslie Wise, Chief of Surgery at Long Island Jewish Hospital on Long Island, read the chapter on breast cancer. I thank him not only for these efforts, but even more for being the rare type of surgeon who guides patients with breast cancer through the haze and helps them select the minor or major procedure with which they will be the most comfortable.

Thanks, too, to the late Dr. Martin B. Levene, Deputy Director, Joint Center for Radiation Therapy at Harvard Medical School, who kindly read the section on radiation therapy for breast cancer.

Thanks to Vicki Fretz, and especially to Michele Cahill French, patients whose letters added a personal touch to the first chapter.

Thanks to Ann Jones, who made editorial rearrangements of the chapters so that they flow as a book. As a physician whose previous longest writing attempts were forty-minute speeches, it was comforting to know that, though the manuscript had to be completed in three-and-a-half months, the final editing could be shared with an accomplished writer.

Last, but not least, many thanks to Elizabeth Scarpelli, who assisted me through the research projects. She also pitched in to type the first, second, and final manuscripts. Her efforts are most gratefully appreciated.

Introduction

My mother never wanted me to go to medical school because she didn't want me to have to work that hard. She wanted me to be a wife and a mother. I followed that advice, but I also went to medical school. She is proud of me, but she still tells me that I work too hard and should lie down and rest in the afternoon.

I grew up in a small town in upstate New York and never even realized that I should be "liberated." My medical school made sure I understood that I had taken some man's place and that I was duly appreciative. I did my work, never rocked the boat, and learned what I was taught. I married at the end of my third year in medical school (at 22, I could no longer afford to be an old maid). I had two children, taking off only a few weeks from my practice after each was born. Besides running a practice, I found time to cook, bake, and play the piano, and do all the typical things and errands that wives and mothers do. I often kidded my girlfriends that all this kept me out of the department stores, and this made my husband happy.

As time went on, however, and I had more years of practice under my belt, I began to be more and more concerned about medical care, especially medical care for women.

Whether it was the fact that my consciousness was raised or that I was just a late bloomer, I was becoming aware that too often, women were burdened with guilt and blamed for having symptoms just because doctors didn't know how to treat them. Surgeons were all too eager to do surgery, and women were being given all too many tranquilizers and receiving all too little tender loving concern from their doctors.

I began to feel that women would never have better health care unless they themselves pursued it. Without being prodded, the medical community was obviously not going to make any changes itself, and unless women became more educated about their bodies, they would never have the ability to press for change, for they would simply not know enough to be able to make an informed protest. That was where I felt some very special responsibility. As a woman and as a doctor, I felt that I should do whatever I could to improve the situation.

And so I have appeared often on radio and television, given lectures, and now written this book—all to get into the hands of women the information they need to secure better personal care.

There is good news in women's health! There is good news in virtually every aspect of women's health. The catch is that you have to be aware of the new developments and changes, or else the good news may never do you any good.

Women deserve the very best, especially when it comes to health care. But in order to get the very best, you have to know when to wait and see rather than allow yourself to be pushed into unnecessary surgery. It is frequently the case in medicine that less is better than more. As a non-surgeon, my orientation has always been toward treating problems medically rather than surgically whenever possible. To resort to surgery, in many instances, is to admit that we don't know how to treat a disease medically; and in many cases, surgery should only be the last resort. Yet women are too often subjected to unnecessary and dangerous surgical procedures. You should not let yourself be coaxed or coerced into the operating room; but, on the other hand, you must be able to assess the telltale signs that indicate that you really *need* surgery, and the sooner the better.

To be able to know the difference, you must be medically informed. Every women must take the responsibility for the decisions that concern her health care. Too often a woman faces the prospect of making these decisions without any real scientific understanding. Worse, sometimes when questioning major gynecologic decisions, she is faced with a physician who smugly says, "Are you challenging my judgment?" Don't be intimidated. The doctor is not your father, and you are no longer a little girl. He is performing a service that you are paying him for. If you are not getting what you want, find another doctor and don't let him make you feel guilty about it. This book will give you the information you need to help you in your decision making.

(Incidentally, you will notice that throughout this book I refer to the doctor as "he." There are many women doctors [9 percent], and I am sure we will see more and more women entering the profession. But the fact is that most doctors are male, and more important, the whole orientation of the medical profession is masculine.)

It always saddens me to hear how often women simply bury their heads in the sand and passively accept whatever treatment a doctor doles out to them. Too often, they fail even to participate in making a treatment decision because they are overwhelmed by the situation and by their complete lack of knowledge. These women are not stupid. On the contrary, often they are lawyers, engineers, and accountants. Yet they docilely accept any prescription for health care— swallowing powerful drugs with dangerous side effects, even submitting their bodies to the surgical knife—all with scarcely a question asked; though they would never dream of abdicating control over their lives to such an extent to a car salesman or a realtor, or even a boss. It has always baffled me that a woman will battle her interior decorator tooth and claw for the right to keep a stringy philodendron but never question a doctor's advice that she get rid of her uterus.

Who is to blame? I think that there is quite enough blame to be spread around. The women of my generation were brought up to be shy and reticent about matters that concerned their bodies, especially their sexual organs. Mothers generally understand too little to be able to explain most body functions to their daughters. Schools and health classes avoid emotional or sexual subjects and stay properly boring by only covering the most academic areas of body function. And physicians certainly haven't been much help in expanding our understanding about our bodies. Many of them offer enlightenment in medical jargon so that their explanations are nonunderstandable and condescending. We are all to blame. We are all, therefore, also victims.

And so, with a passive female patient population, a male-dominated medical profession has long cast a male bias over women's health care, with the result that we have too many hysterectomies, radical mastectomies, and other unnecessary surgery being performed on women. Paradoxically, these rates are highest in the United States, where some of the world's most sophisticated, educated, and feminist women live. It is time to challenge some of the "eternal truths" that have come down to us through years of male medical care. It is time to open our eyes and see the situation as it really exists. It is time to challenge complacency, armed with new knowledge.

I am not a renegade. Rather, I have chosen to fight for better women's health care from within the medical system. I have published research articles in major medical journals. I am a Clinical Associate Professor of Family Medicine at the State University of New York at Stony Brook. I am past president of the two-hundred-member (nearly 100 percent male) Nassau County Academy of Family Practice, serve on the board of directors of the American Cancer Society, and have spoken in many countries about my research, as well as on radio and TV across the United States. I am trying from within the medical profession. Now it is your turn. You must try from the outside, from the patient's side.

As you go through the first chapter, you will realize that it's not your fault if you suffer from menstrual pain. There is a chemical basis for menstrual pain, and women who suffer from it are neither neurotic nor weak.

Women who have suffered in silence and guilt no longer need hide their pain from the rest of the world, for there is now scientific proof that they don't suffer because they are "mental cases." Physicians and society have always looked askance at women suffering with menstrual pain; and women have been duped into obediently believing that their errant psyches were to blame for this malady. Physicians have preferred to take this approach rather than admit that they didn't know how to treat this problem, and at the same time were unwilling to undertake significant research on it. Now the good news for women with menstrual cramps is that there are nonnarcotic, nonhormonal, nonsedating medications that can be taken for pain beginning with the onset of flow.

Premenstrual tension is another area in which there has been virtually no research. I have just completed a study using drugs known as antiprostaglandins to alleviate premenstrual symptoms, and as far as I know, it is the only such study in the world! So far, no overall cure for all the symptoms of premenstrual distress has been found, but some very simple changes in diet will get rid of most symptoms in most women. To date, however, the symptoms of irritability, bloating, breast tenderness, lethargy, and weight gain have been mostly ignored or treated with inappropriate medication.

Another area that I have researched is estrogen-replacement therapy. The medical community has blindly treated menopause by using any remedy currently in vogue. In the fifties, women were treated with tranquilizers; in the sixties, with estrogen; and in the seventies, all estrogen was taken away and we came full circle back to Valium. Many women are currently denied estrogen by their physicians, or they are afraid to take it.

Estrogen can cause an increase in the incidence of endometrial cancer,* especially if it is used incorrectly. Unfortunately, most doctors in the United States, in my estimation, use estrogen incorrectly. Estrogen-replacement therapy, coupled with replacement of the second female hormone, progesterone, can be safe and may even result in lower rates of endometrial cancer than usually occur in untreated women. And, properly administered, estrogen-progesterone therapy may actually help prevent bone loss, atrophic vaginitis, and coronary heart disease—menopausal complaints that cause more suffering and death than endometrial cancer does.

This book also discusses breast cancer and its detection and treatment. It is now abundantly clear that survival rates are little affected by the type of breast surgery that is performed. Minimal breast surgery with preservation of the breast, in conjunction with postoperative radiation, is a choice that most women with early breast cancer can elect. As far as I am concerned, there should be *no more radical mastectomies.* And early detection methods, such as breast self-examination and mammography, make possible lesser surgical procedures and higher survival rates.

Contraception has always been women's responsibility, but these days there are more methods to choose from—intrauterine devices, spermicides, diaphragms, pills, female sterilization, and that good old standby, the condom. Vasectomy can bring responsibility for birth control back to the male and save a woman from dangerous drugs or major surgical procedures. Physicians, however, seem to prefer to put the responsibility—and the risks—on women, so the least you can do is study your options.

So many unnecessary hysterectomies are performed in this country every day; it is time women know that they can choose to keep their bodies intact. Many uterine conditions

---

*Cancer of the lining of the uterus.

that supposedly "call for" hysterectomy can be treated with medication or lesser procedures, and conditions which doctors call precancerous do not necessarily lead to cancer at all. At the very least, women need a specific diagnosis (which this book will help you interpret) and a second opinion before considering hysterectomy.

I love my patients too much to deny them their right to medical choice, and I have written this book because I believe that patients should know enough to be able to choose. Unlike some of my male colleagues, I feel no need to impress or intimidate my patients. I do not have to be in a position of absolute authority. I want my patients to know and understand as much as possible about their conditions and the various options for treatment, and to reach their own informed decisions. In the long run, it is better for all of us. I am able to share some of my responsibility, and they—being well informed and in control of their lives— are relieved of the fear and anxiety of being helpless. I think it's okay if we lean on each other a little. And my patients seem to think so, too.

"Love" may seem to be a funny word to use in a discussion of doctors and patients, but I sincerely feel that doctors need to love their patients. If a doctor really feels concern for a patient, then he will always treat the patient to the best of his ability. The patient will always come before his own personal considerations. The physician's ego or macho behavior or financial self-interest must not be allowed to influence care. The physician should think first of the patient, second of himself. That, to me, is the definition of "love" in medicine. Indeed, thinking of others first is love in any relationship. The medical-school curriculum needs to add a little of this to its lectures.

About four months after my research on menstrual pain had been published, my teenage daughter stuck her head into my consultation room and said, "Mommy, I have cramps."

I looked up at her, and she made a funny face at me and rubbed her tummy. I smiled back and took a capsule from a bottle near my desk.

"Come into the kitchen with me, Cindy. You have to take this with a glass of milk."

I poured the milk, then took the capsule and placed it in her hand. As I did so, I was suddenly struck by the full significance that moment held for me. I had spent three years proving that this drug, taken one or two days each month, could banish monthly menstrual pain. It had been worth every moment. For now I could stand in my kitchen with an arm around my daughter and hand her the gift of a small capsule that could literally guarantee that she would never have to suffer. She swallowed the capsule and drank the milk. I kissed her, realizing that, for her and her generation, life would be free of "the curse" and the mythology that had burdened women through all the ages since Eve. Now and forever more, there would be No More Menstrual Cramps.

And so I give you *No More Menstrual Cramps and Other Good News*.

No More Menstrual Cramps
and Other Good News

CHAPTER 1
No More Menstrual Cramps

I was 16 years old and a freshman at the University of Wisconsin. I was glad the wind was blowing because it meant I could walk bent forward, as if leaning into the wind, so no one would suspect that I couldn't straighten up. My face was freezing from the icy gusts, by my stomach was boiling in pain. I felt as if gravity had increased fifty times and was trying to pull the contents of my abdomen out from between my legs.

Why hadn't I picked a school with a smaller campus? I had to endure the pain long enough to walk to the ladies' room in Bascom Hall. That was a twenty-minute walk from my class at the far side of the campus; and from there, it was another twenty-minute walk to my residence. At Bascom Hall, three flights of stairs separated me from the cot in the ladies' room. I knew I had a better chance of making the three flights to the cot than the twenty-minute walk to my dorm, so I literally pulled myself up the stairs, using my arms to raise my legs for the last flight. At last, I slowly let my body down onto the cot, feeling certain that any sudden movement would break my stomach in half, and curled myself up into a silent ball, coat and all. After half an hour, the pain had subsided somewhat, so I got up and trudged the rest of the way home. When I reached the dorm, I was exhausted.

That was twenty years ago, and I still remember it clearly. I had been experiencing dysmenorrhea—menstrual cramps. I didn't expect anybody to be particularly sympathetic. They would have been, I suppose, if I'd had colitis or some other medically "respectable" malady. Menstrual cramps were, I knew, strictly a female problem.

Later, I was to learn that the medical word for women's painful monthly bleeding, "dysmenorrhea," is Greek. Symptoms vary but include cramping in the lower abdomen, backache, and pain and pulling in the area of the inner thighs. Often these symptoms are accompanied by nausea, vomiting, diarrhea, dizziness, fainting, headache, and flushes of warmth and cold. The pain is usually worst on the first or second day of flow.

There are two types of dysmenorrhea: primary and secondary. In primary dysmenorrhea, pelvic examination reveals no physical abnormality to account for the pain. Secondary dysmenorrhea, on the other hand, is caused by an organic problem such as endometriosis, fibroids, cancer, polyps, IUDs, or other gynecologic difficulties. For obvious reasons, the discussions in this book will be confined mainly to primary dysmenorrhea.

The medical profession had never considered menstrual cramps a medical problem of any significance. I don't remember hearing the topic seriously discussed when I was in medical school, although I certainly could have used some information on the subject. I had a terrible time every month. It wasn't just the cramps; the nausea, vomiting, and diarrhea that came with the pain were almost too much to handle on days when hospital rounds started at 5 A.M. and ended after midnight. At that time, there wasn't much to alleviate the pain. And my medical education had taught me only that women who suffered were hysterical.

When I was a first-year medical student, I decided to see a gynecologist. After examining me, he sat me down to talk to me "like a father." The best thing I could do to get rid of my monthly pain, he said, would be to have a baby.

I told him thanks, but I had three and a half more years of medical school left, and besides, I wasn't married—in fact, I didn't even have a boyfriend. But to him, I was not a person with particular goals and needs; I was just another female. He still thought that having a baby was the best idea for every woman with menstrual pain but condescended to treat me with some pills that I had to take for twenty-one days each month.

The medication seemed to work fine, and after renewing the bottle each month for a year, I returned for a checkup. When he asked me how I was doing, I replied, "Fine, my cramps are gone."

"Yes," he said, "those birth-control pills really can do wonders."

I gasped. "Birth-control pills? Is that what they were?"

He looked at me incredulously. "What did you think they were?"

"I really had no idea what they were, but I never expected that you would give *me* birth-control pills."

When I got home and over my surprise, I thought the entire episode was very funny. Here I was, a medical student, and I had been on birth-control pills for a year and never knew it. Birth-control pills were very new then, and like all other prescriptions were put in bottles with prescription numbers, but no drug names. I was a typical female patient of the sixties. No matter that I was a medical student; I just took what the doctor gave me, never questioned, and dared not complain.

As the years went by, the doctor's advice that having children would alleviate my menstrual pain was proved incorrect. I accepted my predicament as I always had. Menstrual pain, like the pain of childbirth, was not something I anxiously held in my mind from one episode to the next. As most other women do, I simply forgot about it. Menstrual pain had always been my lot in life—the one unfortunate aspect of being a woman—and I accepted it.

Having become a doctor myself, however, I had learned

of a medication called Edrisal, and I was eager to share the relief it offered with other women. When I asked my patients about their menstrual pain, though, some of them were very surprised that I was interested. Apparently many of them had also learned to grin and bear it. As time went on, I became more and more convinced that menstrual pain was a significant problem, at least in my practice.

My opportunity to explore the scope of the problem—and, not so incidentally, to raise my consciousness—came when I was asked to be a keynote speaker in April 1976 at a symposium on "Women in Industry," presented jointly by Stony Brook University and South Oaks Hospital on Long Island. My assigned topic was "Unique Health Problems of Women in Industry." By that time, I was teaching residents in family medicine at the State University of New York Medical School at Stony Brook, and I had often spoken at women's meetings on such topics as contraception and menopause. I was not especially well informed about industrial health problems, but since I had taken care of women in my private practice for the past twelve years, I was pretty sure that whatever affected their physical well-being would affect their job performance as well.

I decided that my audience of five hundred professional people—physicians, educators, labor leaders, and career women—were going to hear about menstrual pain. I knew from my practice that menstrual pain was very real and not, as so many doctors said, a psychological problem. And I knew that it heavily affected job performance and the physical and mental well-being of an enormous number of women. It *was* important.

I spent a great deal of time preparing my forty-minute presentation. I worked weekends, reading up on the areas I was going to discuss. The more research I did, the more perturbed and resentful I became, because there was almost nothing on the subject of dysmenorrhea in the American scientific literature.

The many gynecology textbooks I went through contained no scientific data. Dysmenorrhea was presented as a purely psychological disorder, although its cause could not be adequately explained. In desperation, I even resorted to popular books full of menstrual mythology and taboos. It was interesting to know that there were still menstrual huts in darkest Africa, and that menstruating women were thought to cause crops to die, wine to go sour, and dogs to go mad, but this was hardly the type of data to present before five hundred professionals who were expecting to hear about "Women in Industry."

I began to wonder why there was so little real scientific data on menstrual cramps and why all the medical literature—what little there was of it—laid the cause to women's psyches. I had had menstrual pain since the age of 16, and I was pretty confident that I was not neurotic. Menstrual cramps often awakened me from a sound sleep at 4 A.M. Certainly, if I were as hysterical as all the literature postulated, I could have picked a more convenient time for my cramps, such as the middle of a busy afternoon with all my phones ringing and all my patients complaining of long waits in the reception room.

The morning before my speech, I mentioned to a woman labor relations expert who would be attending the symposium that I would be talking about menstrual pain. She glared at me and then said threateningly, "It's a major problem, but you mustn't talk about, because there's no solution. It's a constant threat to our survival and advancement in industry. You'll ruin it for all of us!"

I was somewhat taken aback but managed to reply, "It's no good to continue to sweep the problem under the rug. It's time to face it and find some kind of solution." But we were both aware that the male establishment and, by extension, the business world branded women who suffered from dysmenorrhea as second-class citizens. What better excuse could there be for excluding women from executive positions in business or government? How could a woman who was regularly incapacitated due to menstrual problems be depended upon to function optimally at all times? How could a person requiring a narcotic analgesic each month be expected to function well physically and to exercise good judgment?

In my intensive research and reading, however, I had come across two short papers, one prepared by A. Schwartz, U. Zor, H. R. Lindner, and S. Naor in Israel in 1974[1] and the other by V. R. Pickles in England in 1972.[2] Both presented evidence to explain why women experienced menstrual pain, and both offered the promise of scientific treatment.

It was as if someone had suddenly illuminated a dark and mysterious closet, and for the first time, I could plainly see what was in it.

I had spent four years in medical school, completed an internship, and practiced medicine for twelve years, but somehow I had never before been quite so aware of the smugness of the medical community regarding this problem. I began to get angry: it was clear that dysmenorrhea had been labeled a psychological problem just because no one seemed to care enough to investigate whether it had a physiologic basis. What was still being taught in medical schools could not be reconciled with the new information I had found. And in the face of the evidence that dysmenorrhea does have a physical cause, the familiar label "hysteria" seemed particularly ugly and the time-honored treatment of referring patients to psychiatrists particularly cruel. There was a real reason for menstrual cramps—and there was definitely the possibility of a real cure.

At the time I addressed the symposium, I was just becoming aware of the enormity of the suffering as well as the tremendous amount of lost work hours that dysmenorrhea caused, and the prejudice against women that this absenteeism created. I kept thinking of all the women patients whose suffering I had tried to help and all the data on the national extent of suffering that I had unearthed in the last few weeks. Dysmenorrhea is the most common cause of lost work and school hours in the United States, accounting for 140 million lost working hours each year.

So it is hardly surprising that some labor unions, in their reluctance to accept women into their ranks, have embraced the notion that women can never function adequately in the work force because of this feminine handicap, and that days lost because of menstrual problems are a sore spot with employers as well as with unions.

Of the 75 million women in the United States who menstruate, nearly half have menstrual discomfort with some regularity. Of these, approximately 10 percent, or 3.5 million women, are *completely* incapacitated for one to two days each month because of pain. It seemed hard to believe that a problem of such magnitude could go on for so long without prompting some interest among medical researchers.

One possible explanation is that the myths society has foisted off on women have made a similar impact on the medical establishment. Since half of the women don't suffer menstrual cramps, doctors are all too willing to blame those who do for bringing on their own illness.

When we were little girls, our mothers taught us that when we first had our periods, we should be good little soldiers and not make a fuss. Many of us had cramps, but we gritted our teeth and suffered in silence lest we be thought of as weak or, even worse, immature. Those of us who continued to experience painful menstruation as we grew up began to hear that our pain was psychological, caused by our dissatisfaction with our lot as women; or that we were malingerers; mollycoddled by our mothers; or hysterical; or else that we suffered from penis envy.

We have become so acculturated to think of dysmenorrhea as a failing that even feminists have difficulty coming to grips with the realities of female physiology. If feminists concerned with achieving male-female equality choose to ignore the problem of incapacitating dysmenorrhea, imagine how easy it is for a medical student to believe that dysmenorrhea is not a serious problem but merely a psychological phenomenon to be obliterated with narcotics and tranquilizers. The gynecology textbooks that medical students read all reinforce the psychological theme. In fact, the men who wrote the textbooks seem to have taken many of their thoughts from the men who wrote the Bible.

Consider the following quotations from well-known gynecology textbooks published between 1952 and 1978:

1952
Novak and Novak, *Textbook of Gynecology*[3]

While many women suffer no discomfort whatsoever during menstruation, a moderate amount of pelvic heaviness and even an occasional cramp may be considered as within normal limits.

It needs no more than a knowledge of human nature to justify the statement that the same degree of peripheral stimulation which in the well balanced, phlegmatic individual will be expressed as a moderate discomfort, *will manifest itself in the high-strung supersensitive girl by severe and incapacitating pain.*

The psychogenic element ... may accentuate the subjective element in a particular case. Among these are a *congenitally unstable and high-strung nervous system, psychic trauma, especially when related to the menstrual periods, and wrong ideas as to the significance and normality of the menstrual function.* This last named factor is frequently encountered by many a young girl at the beginning of her menstrual life when she is *coddled by an overly anxious mother* into the belief that menstruation is a time when she should consider herself unwell. To such a girl, especially if reared in a household where one or more women suffer from dysmenorrhea, *the transition to menstrual invalidism is a very easy one.* [Emphasis added.]

1961
Brewer, *Textbook of Gynecology*[4]

Psychogenic causes are the most common and the most important in cases of primary dysmenorrhea.

It is common that a mother, *who herself is not adjusted,* transmits to her daughter the feeling that menstruation is a period of being unwell. *Menstruation also lends itself as an excuse for avoiding things that are undesired.* In most girls, menstruation is associated with great anxiety, fear and uncertainty. *If an individual happens to be unstable emotionally, these are all enhanced. Most reaction could be obviated by proper counseling prior to puberty.* The individual who does the counseling under ordinary circumstances should not be the mother, older friends, or girls of her own age, but should be a physician. Additional necessary help might be obtained by the use of trained psychologists. This would reduce the frequency of dysmenorrhea to a large extent.

The threshold for pain varies greatly. Most women have some local pelvic sensation at the time of menstruation. *To some this is interpreted as pain, whereas others are capable of ignoring it completely.* [Emphasis added.]

The above passage was from my own personal copy, well worn from my medical-school days. I don't ever remember reading the passage; I doubt that it was ever assigned. I doubt that any of my professors would have found the subject worth discussing.

1978
Parsons and Sommers, *Gynecology*[5]

One major reason why we understand so little of the underlying cause of dysmenorrhea is that we have come to consider it as a psychosomatic illness. No one will deny that the problem has distinct psychiatric overtones. The psychiatric element should not be disregarded for it is well recognized that there is a large psychogenic overlay in most patients who have dysmenorrhea. *It is common to eliminate the pain, but have the patient still be miserable and sullenly resent menstruation because it emphasizes the feminine role which she either doesn't want to take on, or is incapable of.* To the inexperienced adolescent girl, painful cramps may be interpreted as "punishment" for sexual wishes as suggested by Sturgis. It is sometimes a manifestation of retaliation against the dominance of the mother, or it may simply represent a desire to *continue to be a little girl.*

Many reports suggest that *psychotherapy is the sole answer to the problem.* There is no denying the fact that some of these patients present tendencies toward psychosomatic disease and perhaps a lowered threshold for pain. Many girls with severe dysmenorrhea are *perfectly well adjusted to their environment through the rest of the month and rarely seek medical support for other causes.*

They appear perfectly well poised and adjusted after specific therapy but are not improved by placebos.

Apprehensions expressed at the time of the menstrual period may be the result, not the cause of dysmenorrhea. Those who believe that psychic trauma is the basic cause of monthly pain are still *unable to determine which comes first, the pain or the psychogenic response.* [Emphasis added.]

I won't burden you with more learned textbook references to menstrual pain, because they are all pretty much the same. Millions of suffering women have been labeled hysterical even though no one knew the cause of their discomfort, and for the most part, women have meekly accepted that diagnosis.

The men who wrote and read these textbooks trained me and every other physician, and it is difficult for any physician to reject ideas that have been so deeply ingrained. The reaction among nonmedical people is just as biased. Some men may feel sorry for their sisters or wives when they complain, but others whose sisters never experienced a cramp may be confused and impatient when their wives lie in bed clutching a hot-water bottle.

Gym teachers often play the role of villain to many young girls. They are rarely sympathetic and often demand, "Stop babying yourself. Just get up and out there and you'll be fine." Bosses, whether male or female, usually don't appreciate the problem, either. A woman who calls in to say that she has the flu or a migraine gets a sympathetic response: "I hope you feel better soon. Be sure to rest and take care of yourself." But should she confess that she can't come to work because of menstrual cramps, she will hear a long silence at the other end of the wire. Her boss will be positive that she is skipping work to go to a special sale at Macy's or to clean the house for some unexpected company.

Women who do not suffer from cramps tend to have a holier-than-thou attitude toward women who do, considering them overdramatic malingerers who are mentally and physically inferior. They reason, "I'm a woman and I also have a period each month. I don't have pain and I don't complain and carry on, and she shouldn't either." This attitude has been devastating to women experiencing dysmenorrhea. Not only do they suffer, but their own sisters castigate them for doing so.

I received a letter from a patient that I think dramatically illustrates this attitude. She wrote:

Dear Penny,

I never had menstrual cramps. When I was 48, you suggested that I have a uterine biopsy by aspiration method to properly diagnose my bleeding problem. You mentioned that I would probably experience some menstrual-like cramps during the procedure. I was confident that I could handle a little discomfort easily.

Wow! Hell! Damn! What an experience ... found out the little word "cramps" could be aching, gripping, throbbing, piercing pain—like being stabbed internally with a knife that won't quit.

The experience made me reconsider my attitude toward other women and their periodic cramps. In retrospect, I feel badly about my indifference and out-and-out coldness toward their rough and unbearable pain. I can best explain my attitude by citing some flashbacks.

1. One of my first jobs was in the fan-mail department of an ad agency. I recall a woman who took three days of each month off from work. Our superior (a woman) was not only sympathetic but covered for her. I was absolutely furious that Carol had automatic vacations with pay, while I was pushed harder at the office to make up for her absence. I remember she would come back to work and talk about the godawful pain and spending three days in bed with a hot-water bottle and aspirin. My thought was, "I'll bet!" I just wanted her to shut up about her make-believe cramps. After all, if she wanted to be a cheat and a phony, what was it to me.

2. I worked many seasons with a model who once a month pulled a routine that she couldn't possibly wear ten outfits

"this week"; it would be a killer to do five. The designer and manufacturer always took pity on her; she settled for seven and I did thirteen for those days. I felt pure resentment for her pulling a cheap stunt like that while I did double-time, ending up totally exhausted because of this redheaded crybaby!

3. Then there was the relative whose husband and family literally planned their lives around the wife's period. Their response to an invitation to dinner or any social get-together always depended on Mary's precious cycle. I thought Mary had a lousy, negative way of being the center of attention.

How superior I felt in these situations. After all, I never discussed my cycle with anyone and would never let anyone's life be changed a hair just because I happened to be a woman with the *same* monthly inconvenience.

Through all the years of working in many job situations, involvement with community groups, and social encounters, always women like these three would be there somewhere with their "female" complaints. I developed methods of tactfully changing the subject (out of disinterest) and avoiding crampy women altogether.

Now that I know what these women may have been experiencing, I feel sorry that I did not at least give them the benefit of the doubt! Amazing (to discover about myself) that I worked as a telephone counselor for Helpline and really listened to all kinds of human problems and suffering with empathy and some ability to be helpful and reassuring. Yet I could not or would not use this attitude toward women with cramps!

Hope some of my feelings will be helpful to your research.

Vicki

She, like too many other women, could not comprehend the magnitude of the impact dysmenorrhea can have on a sufferer.

One of my patients, a woman named Michele, had led an especially miserable life because of her monthly pain. For her, the catastrophe lasted five days each month. She wrote me a poignant twenty-two-page letter about menstrual pain and the effect it had upon her life. Among many other things, she said:

I started to menstruate when I was 12. The pain did not occur the first few times. The first time it happened I was in the kitchen getting tea for my mother. Suddenly, a terrible pain doubled me over, and I could hardly get my breath. I could not stand straight and when I reached my mother, she told me to sit on my bed, and that it would pass. She was quite nice that time and told me that sometimes it had been bad for her, too. Later on, after a half-year had passed, she was fed up with me. She began to hate my crying and twisting in pain. I was a nuisance, to say the least. Finally, one day when I was thirteen, she told me that if I didn't stop crying that instant, she would walk out on me and leave me alone. I sat there and shuddered, but I didn't make any more noise. My mother made it plain. I learned that I could not cry out or she and other people would withdraw from me.

When I got older, this lesson was reinforced. I could mention my problem once, maybe twice, but then the school nurses and personnel all turned a deaf ear. Teachers would not help me cope; they shook their heads at such absurdity, believing that I had suddenly turned into a goldbrick. They were not about to be fooled. Past history also seemed to count for nothing. I always loved basketball and participated enthusiastically in gym. Once a month, however, I would incur the wrath of my gym teacher who decided that I suddenly just didn't want to improve my basketball skills. Her attitude cooled the attitudes of the girls in my class for me, also. Who would want to associate with such an unreliable person?

My condition also strained my family ties with my sister. My sister was convinced that I should just take Midol for my cramps. Midol? I tried it and could have taken a truckload of the stuff and it wouldn't have made any difference. I also tried all the other over-the-counter products with exactly the same results: none. My sister could not be convinced that Midol was not adequate for my pain. She thought I was faking.

When I was 18, I had a horseback-riding accident in which I broke my back in the middle. The first doctor who examined me failed to X-ray the middle back and said there was nothing wrong but some bruises. I seemed to have too much pain for mere bruises, but since my mother and I had been told officially that I was uninjured, there was nothing for me to do but get on with things the best I could. Two weeks later my father, who did not like the way I was moving, sent me to Knickerbocker Hospital for more X-rays. There they found out that my spine had been broken (in addition to my coccyx) and proceeded to put me in a wheelchair and tell me that I must not take another step, which I thought was pretty funny (except for the pain) because for two weeks I had been walking, cleaning, living on my own, and even hiking in that condition. As you know, Knickerbocker is a busy New York City hospital, used to seeing plenty of the rougher side of life. Yet, that night, the resident who had examined me and taken the X-rays stopped by my room to speak to me. He said, "I just wanted to see how the bravest girl I've ever met is getting along." His kindness surprised me, but so did the fact that he thought my talking calmly, normally, and not crying or fainting with the enormous pain I was in, was surprising. (I should mention that I had had absolutely no pain medication of any kind up to this point because no one had noticed my injuries; nor did I receive or take any during this experience.) The rest of the hospital staff also found my behavior very surprising, as I discovered the next morning.

Bang! the door slammed back. In marched a supervising doctor followed by three residents in single file like ducklings. Without preamble the doctor told me to turn my head sideways on the pillow. I did so, only to have him ram his thumb as hard as he could behind my ear. I just looked at him and blinked, as much out of astonishment as anything else. Whereupon he turned to the residents and said, "There you have it, a classic example of negative reaction to pain." Silently, they turned and marched out as they had come in. So much for being a guinea pig.

There was one thing they did not know, however, about my ability to take pain. It's not that I don't feel it; I have the same number of nerve endings per square foot as anyone else. The difference is that I had been in training for years to endure it. I was used to coping through a haze of nauseating pain, used to having a conversation when every nerve in me was screaming out, used to getting dressed and getting on a bus when I felt as though a red-hot iron was going to knock my stomach out. I got my training every month without fail, when my period came.

I, of course, developed such techniques as I could for enduring this experience, such as mentally talking myself through something, step by step. "Now, just reach your left hand for your other shoe—just hold your breath a minute longer and the pain may ease up for a second." Or, "Just watch the clock, only thirty more minutes till the class bell rings, only twenty-seven more, only twenty more until you can run to the girls' room and close the toilet door and rock back and forth to try and ease the pain, where nobody can see you and sneer at your predicament."

These great techniques were not much. Obviously, they only helped me to endure what I had to endure anyway to live up to our society's conviction that this condition does not exist and need not be remedied.

In addition to her unbearable pain, Michele had to contend with a succession of doctors who couldn't provide any relief for her. In her letter, she described some of her encounters with doctors.

Dr. D., a gynecologist, said that he had seen a few others like me. He didn't know why my pain was so bad, but at least he did not deny that it could possibly be real.

Treatment: Demerol injections and tablets. On the first day he would give me a shot because it took so many tablets to give me relief. He did a D & C, hoping to find that I had endometriosis. Unfortunately, or fortunately, there was none. The pain, however, eased for a few months after the D & C. When things got bad again, he suggested two other surgical procedures. One was a hysterectomy; the other was an operation to cut the nerves in my stomach.

Dr. T., a gynecologist filling in for Dr. D., refused to give me a prescription for Demerol tablets. He said that they were completely unnecessary. He then told my husband that no such severe problems exist. I still resent his smug attitude. I still remember the next few days and the pain that I endured.

Dr. W., a psychiatrist, thought that my parents' divorce was

the cause of my pain even though my pain predated by years
any sign of family trouble.

Dr. G., another gynecologist, said that my tipped uterus was
at fault. He said that there was no need for Demerol. His prescription was to assume a Sphinx-like position twice a day for
fifteen minutes (on hands and knees with rear in the air), so
uterus and muscles would revert to correct position. I tried
this for a while, but it made no difference.

Dr. H.'s treatment: have a baby! He delivered this advice
in a very condescending, patronizing tone. He never inquired
about the security of my marriage or any possible career interests
or aspirations that I might have. Nor did he mention what I
was to do if I had a baby girl who developed her problem
at twelve. Was she supposed to have a baby too?

Dr. I.: The sneering disbelief of his nurse during my physical
exam discouraged me from trying to describe the problem. Later
she would answer my phone calls to the doctor and say, "Really,
Mrs. E., this is quite unnecessary and absurd."

Dr. J.: Tipped uterus at fault. Insert a pessary to untip it
and hold it in place.

About her high rate of narcotic intake during these years,
Michele had this to say.

Demerol was not exactly a good solution, but it was the best
that I could find for some years. I was often nauseated and
dizzy from the drug but at least it got rid of the worst portion
of the pain. Some of the doctors and nurses I met thought
I only wanted the pills for my "drug habit," but I can honestly
say that I never took a single pill except for the pain I had
during menstruation. How could I? I needed them too desperately ever to waste a single one.

Not all women suffer like Michele. Many of those who
did were relieved by the introduction of birth-control pills.
In fact, the pill might well have been the solution for many,
except that after they had been on the market for several
years, their dangerous side effects started coming to light.
Nevertheless, before that discovery, the pill got me through
medical school, my internship, and my early years of practice.

After I had two children, my menstrual pain was somewhat lessened, but it was far from gone. Different symptoms appeared, such as leg achiness, which was sometimes as annoying as the cramping itself. After my second child was born, I went back on the pill, but I wasn't at ease. I knew I couldn't stay on the pill, especially after a doctor friend and I couldn't make up our minds whether an episode of leg tenderness I suffered was caused by phlebitis, a known side effect of the pill.

Now I had two problems: menstrual pain and birth control. My husband and I both felt that I had taken my share of responsibility for birth control throughout our marriage, so he decided it was his turn and had a vasectomy. That solved the birth-control problem, but the menstrual pain remained. I began taking a product called Edrisal that was on the market for dysmenorrhea. It worked well and even was effective on that draggy feeling that often accompanies menstruation. It worked because it contained Benzedrine, a drug best known as the "upper" speed, but which also acts to relax smooth muscles such as those involved in uterine cramps. The other ingredients of Edrisal were aspirin and phenacetin. The drug did have some minor side effects; I would take only half a tablet at a time because a larger dose made me jittery; and sometimes the patients for whom I prescribed it didn't sleep very well. But it did get rid of most of the cramps.

Then, quite suddenly, Edrisal was taken off the market because it contained Benzedrine and because it was a combination drug—that is, a drug made up of more than one ingredient. Medical thinking at the time held that all drugs should be dispensed separately, never together, so that the doctor could adjust the amount of one drug before he added a second. This idea still persists but has often backfired because patients do not like to take two or three separate pills when just one would do. Moreover, patients often forget to take them all. As so often happens, medical thinking has reversed itself, and combinations are creeping back into use again.

But Edrisal is gone. I still remember the day the drug detail man told me that it would no longer be available. My reaction was, "Oh my God, are there any bottles left anywhere?" There were, and I got two 100-tablet bottles. I rationed them out so sparingly to my patients and myself that there are still some left somewhere in the bottom of one of my drug cabinets. And I still wonder if the people who forced Edrisal off the market knew the misery they caused.

It was just about this time that I was asked to address the conference on "Women in Industry" and began reading up on my chosen topic. Now that birth-control pills were coming under fire and Edrisal was no longer available, I had a real stake in trying to understand menstrual pain, why it occurred, and how it might be helped. There had to be some hope somewhere, but it certainly was not in the gynecology textbooks. But I found that hope—the good news for women with dysmenorrhea—buried in the scientific-research literature under the heading: prostaglandins.

Prostaglandins were first noted in the scientific-research literature in 1930, when Drs. Kurzrok and Lieb discovered that substances in human semen caused contraction of strips of uterine muscle. This contraction-causing substance was named prostaglandin because traces of it had been found in specimens from the prostate gland as well as the seminal vesicles (both of which are male reproductive glands). In 1957, Pickles suggested that excess prostaglandin in menstrual fluid may cause dysmenorrhea. In 1961, there was only one article in the literature about prostaglandins. In 1962, the exact structure of two groups of prostaglandins was discovered. In 1964, prostaglandins were first biosynthesized in research laboratories, and by 1968, prostaglandins were synthesized from relatively inexpensive materials. As the ability to understand prostaglandin chemistry unfolded, the literature literally exploded. By 1972, over two thousand articles were appearing annually.

Early observations seemed to indicate that prostaglandins

played a limited role in body chemistry, since they were thought to be unique to the prostate gland or reproductive system. But later research revealed that prostaglandins are to be found in nearly every cell of the body. They are derived from the essential unsaturated fatty acids in the diet which undergo a series of enzymatic reactions to form prostaglandins.

Most prostaglandins are not hormones. Hormones, by definition, are produced in one organ and go through the bloodstream to exert their effect on a second distant organ. For example, hormones manufactured in the pituitary gland within the brain tell the thyroid how hard to work. The thyroid, in turn, produces its own hormones and sends them back to the brain via the bloodstream in increasing concentration. The increased level of thyroid hormone then instructs the pituitary gland to turn off so that the thyroid, in turn, can discontinue production.

Prostaglandins are different in that they usually act where they are produced. Prostaglandins regulate the tone of smooth muscles, the nonvoluntary muscles of the body. We cannot voluntarily control these muscles—the muscles of the blood vessels, the uterus, and the intestines, for example— as we can control the muscles in our arms and legs that we command to contract to help us walk and work. Smooth muscles cause uterine contractions, change blood vessel diameter, and regulate intestinal activity—all without our conscious control. Smooth muscles are controlled, to some extent, by prostaglandin activity; and fluctuations in prostaglandin levels and ratios cause the muscles to react in different ways. The final effect of prostaglandins on smooth-muscle tissue depends not only on the total amount of prostaglandins present, but also on the *ratio* of different kinds of prostaglandins present. This ratio is critical, because one type of prostaglandin may cause smooth muscle to relax while another causes it to contract.

The uterine lining produces two prostaglandins, prostaglandin E and prostaglandin F (nine groups have been identified so far, dubbed A through I). Their levels increase as the time of menstruation approaches. The highest levels occur at the onset of flow. Prostaglandin F probably causes a greater increase in muscle tone and contraction of the uterus than prostaglandin E. When prostaglandins are produced in excess amounts or F is in excess of E, the uterus is overactive and contracts too much, causing cramps and pain. The uterus squeezes so hard that it compresses the uterine blood vessels and cuts off the blood supply. This situation is very much like what occurs in the heart when its blood supply is cut off by a clot or blood vessel spasm during a heart attack. The heart also is a muscle, and when it suffers a decrease in its blood supply, the pain (angina) is excruciating. The result is the same in both instances: pain occurs when a muscle does not have sufficient oxygen because the blood flow has been cut off. The pain of dysmenorrhea is analogous to the pain experienced during a heart attack. Perhaps dysmenorrhea would have been better understood if it had been named uterine angina.

And if that were not enough, some of the excess prostaglandin escapes from the uterus and into the bloodstream, where it may affect other smooth muscles in the body before it is destroyed. The smooth muscle of the gut is stimulated and contracts too rapidly and propels food along too quickly, causing diarrhea. The smooth muscle in blood vessels may cause blood vessels to constrict and dilate. That's why some women feel cold and hot flashes. And some women will faint because a sudden dilation of the blood vessels causes a pooling of blood in their legs and feet, depriving the brain of blood and oxygen.

Dr. Pickles was very much aware of the tie between dysmenorrhea and prostaglandins. In his article in *Nature* in 1972, he wrote:

> The fact that anovulatory cycles [menstrual cycles during which no egg is produced] (normally pain-free) in one young subject ended with menstrual losses having only one-fifth the usual content of prostaglandin-like material was reported briefly in 1967.

In other words, as far back as 1967, it was known that women who had menstrual pain had five times the amount of prostaglandin in their menstrual fluid as did women who were without pain. Even earlier, in 1965, Pickles had reported that there were evident differences in the prostaglandin content of menstrual fluid between women with dysmenorrhea and those who were "normal."[6]

Pickles also suggested the possibility of specific drug treatment. In his 1972 article in *Nature,* he wrote:

> One of the anti-inflammatory drugs could possibly prove to be of value in dysmenorrhea, which may be associated with abnormal prostaglandin action, especially as aspirin has commonly been recommended for its simple treatment.

Speaking of indomethacin, a specific anti-inflammatory drug being used for the treatment of arthritis in England at that time, he noted that "The concentration of prostaglandin ... shown to be high in women with dysmenorrhea ... is lowered by indomethacin treatment."

But Pickles was not the first person to suggest a cure for menstrual pain in the literature. As early as 1953, an article by W. W. Fox in the prestigious English medical journal the *Lancet* reported on the value of phenylbutazone (another anti-inflammatory drug) in treating menstrual pain.[7] More recently, in a letter to the *British Medical Journal,* G. G. Hill wrote:

> In 1973 ... you published a letter from me stating that for several years I had successfully treated most cases of dysmenorrhea with indomethacin [Indocin] ... I had in fact mentioned this on more than one occasion to the representatives of the makers, but without apparent interest on the firm's part.[8]

Imagine! In 1973, Hill had an effective cure for menstrual pain, but no one cared. And women continued to suffer— even though several researchers had written about curing menstrual pain with anti-inflammatory drugs, and many of these drugs were already used worldwide for other purposes. The English researchers had constantly referred to dysmenorrhea as a physiologic problem. Here was the first written material I found that did not refer to dysmenorrhea as a hysterical problem of complaining women.

But even in England, where so much of this background research had been conducted, the drug companies didn't think dysmenorrhea was important or that a medication to get rid of it would be worth researching. Women were destined to suffer; it served us right. After all, Eve ate the forbidden apple in the Garden of Eden, and the Bible says that, in consequence, we will bring forth our children in pain. And so at least many physicians act as if pain is our due and getting rid of it is almost sacrilegious.

As I continued my studies, I came upon an important and informative paper by Doctors A. Schwartz, U. Zor, H. R. Lindner, and S. Naor, who had collaborated on dysmenorrhea research in Israel. Since their paper is so significant, I want to present here a simplified summary of the original that appeared in the *Journal of Obstetrics/Gynecology* in 1974.

Primary dysmenorrhea is one of the commonest gynecologic complaints and represents a major cause of lost working and school days, yet its pathogenesis remains obscure. No consistently effective treatment has been devised, other than the use of oral contraceptives, a choice that is not always acceptable. Prostaglandins may play a role in the causation of this syndrome. Our studies show that prostaglandin manufacture increases after ovulation.

Excessive release of prostaglandins during menstrual breakdown of the lining of the uterus could lead to painful uterine contraction. Absorption of prostaglandins into the circulation could also account for the diarrhea and weakness that are commonly associated with dysmenorrhea. While this hypothesis still rests on tenuous ground, the clinical pilot trial reported here would seem to lend it some support.

The studies of Vane[9] established that many nonsteroidal anti-inflammatory drugs such as indomethacin, aspirin, and the fenamates are potent inhibitors of the manufacture of prostaglandin.

The fenamates are peculiar in that not only do they inhibit the manufacture of prostaglandin, but they also stop its action on smooth muscle.

Sixteen women with severe dysmenorrhea were in the trial. They were given flufenamic acid (Flunalgan—manufactured in Jerusalem) four times a day, then three times a day for the second and third day of their menses. Treatment with flufenamic acid abolished the symptoms of dysmenorrhea, diarrhea and nausea in all sixteen patients in the thirty-one menstrual periods that were treated. All sixteen patients had their symptoms reappear after the medication was stopped. Treatment of the same group of patients with placebo or tranquilizers afforded no significant relief.

The results of the pilot study showed that treatment with flufenamic acid was extremely effective in relieving the symptoms of dysmenorrhea. . . . Psychogenic factors may play a part in the development of this syndrome, but the negative results obtained in our patients when treated with placebos indicates that relief reported by the patients treated with flufenamic acid was not due to suggestion, but to a specific action for the drug.

Aspirin has traditionally been included in many formulations of medication for dysmenorrhea. Aspirin is an inhibitor of prostaglandin manufacture, but is only partially effective, if at all, in relieving severe dysmenorrhea. The greater efficacy of flufenamic acid is probably due to its ability to stop the manufacture of prostaglandin, as well as to neutralize the activity of preformed prostaglandin so that it cannot cause muscle contraction and pain.[10]

I was overwhelmed by the good news in this paper. Yet although it had been published in 1974, two years earlier, no one seemed to have paid it any attention. Even worse, I was unable to find any follow-up on that study. Larger numbers of patients were needed, along with more sophisticated data. Why hadn't the Israelis done another study that was somewhat better controlled and more scientific to document their findings?

All my research into the problem of dysmenorrhea only exposed a staggering neglect of a crucial area of women's health. When I finally delivered my presentation to the sym-

posium on "Women in Industry" on April 8, 1976, I was
angry. In part, here is what I said:

> Our male-oriented society has never come to grips with men-
> struation. Since antiquity problems and pain related to men-
> struation have been regarded by many physicians as unimportant,
> a sign of woman's weakness, either mental or physical. Even
> today the most common treatment prescribed is to go home,
> stay in bed, and the pains will go away. Or perhaps they will
> go away after you have a baby, or two, but surely they will
> go away when you become menopausal. After all, it doesn't
> last forever.
>
> It is curious that in this day and age when we are probing
> outer space that we permit more than half the population of
> the world to suffer from dysmenorrhea. In 1974 there were
> only eight articles dealing with dysmenorrhea in the entire
> world's literature. In the February 1975 edition of the journal
> *Practitioner,* a leading obstetrician-gynecologist decreed, "En-
> courage a disregard of the pain and encourage a carrying on
> of normal activity."
>
> If it were possible to wave a magic wand and cause some
> of our male colleagues to experience a period or two, the amount
> of research on dysmenorrhea would increase geometrically. We
> all know of the intense research effort that created the birth-
> control pill. One can hypothesize that this research satisfied
> a male goal and, at the same time, made contraception a female
> responsibility. Researching dysmenorrhea satisfies no male goal
> and may even be counterproductive. Why destroy the proof
> that women are the weaker sex?. . .
>
> What little research has been done to date has shown that
> dysmenorrhea has a physiological etiology. This has taken some
> of the onus from women's shoulders. Women do not have men-
> strual cramps because they are hysterical, but because they have
> five times the amount of prostaglandin as women who are rel-
> atively symptom-free. At last there is something that can be
> documented that shows a physiological difference between the
> fortunate women who do not suffer, and those who do. . . .
>
> Drugs that inhibit prostaglandin activity are currently being
> evaluated. Flunalgan (flufenamic acid), an Israeli drug, has the
> ability to neutralize prostaglandin, as well as to prevent its con-
> tinued synthesis. It abolished the symptoms of dysmenorrhea

in 100 percent of the women to whom it was given. Drugs available in this country include Indocin (indomethacin), which is normally used to treat arthritis. This drug also works as a prostaglandin inhibitor. Aspirin is sometimes helpful in dysmenorrhea, and it now seems that its basis for action lies in the fact that it is a partially effective inhibitor of prostaglandin. . . .

The modern physician must take the problem of dysmenorrhea seriously. He must learn to treat this condition appropriately without sedating women out of the job market.[11]

When I finished my speech, I received a long ovation. The topics I discussed—especially dysmenorrhea—had up to then been totally avoided, so that my audience was grateful for any information. "Why haven't we ever heard about this before?" they asked, and in the next breath: "Can you tell us more?" But I had told them all I knew.

By then, however, I was convinced that the problem could be treated with a simple antiprostaglandin medication, but I felt the theory had to be tested further. I was a clinician, not a researcher. I ran a family practice out of a five-room office attached to my home on Long Island. It was the kind of office where my dog was likely to scratch on the office door and be let in by a patient. Often my kids could be heard asking what was for lunch and could I get it for them. It really wasn't the kind of ivory tower that one thinks a researcher should work in.

But I was optimistic. If I could try some flufenamic acid and if it worked, lots of women, including me, would be rid of those monthly cramps. In addition, the terrible guilt that had been laid squarely on the shoulders of women could be lifted.

Setting out to find flufenamic acid, I made a number of phone calls and finally learned that it was manufactured by Warner-Lambert. Dr. Roberts in the international division of Warner-Lambert generously took the time to listen to me. He told me that while flufenamic acid was in use in Europe, the drug was not available in the United States; but he came up with an idea.

"There is a drug related to flufenamic acid in the United States called Ponstel,"* he said. "It is in the same fenamate family of drugs, and both are nonsteroid anti-inflammatories. Ponstel has been on the market for pain since 1967 here in the United States and all over the world. Call Parke-Davis, our domestic company that manufactures the drug, and try your luck."

I felt like Sherlock Holmes. My first order of business was not to call Parke-Davis but my favorite pharmacist. "Send over ten Ponstel capsules, please," I said. More than willing to be the guinea pig for my experiment, I could hardly wait for my next period. At the first sign, I took the first capsule and waited. I didn't have any pain. Four hours later, I began to be uncomfortable. Were these my first cramps, or had the capsule taken away the early pains? I took another. After about half an hour, my cramps subsided. It was almost too good to be true. I couldn't discern any side effects. I wasn't sleepy and my head was clear. At the end of twenty-four hours, I had taken just four capsules. I decided to try it for another month. After all, I had to be sure that I had not talked myself into believing that the medication worked just because I wanted it to.

The next month, on the first day of my menses, I was scheduled for hospital-clinic teaching duty in a large hospital with corridors that seemed to go on for miles. All of us who taught there joked about needing roller skates even on our good days; and on those days when my legs felt like they weighed a ton each, walking became a formidable challenge. I took a Ponstel when the flow began. The day came and went. The Ponstel had made two distinct differences: I had no cramps and my legs didn't ache.

Now I was sure that the drug worked—at least for me. The next morning I called Dr. Petrick, a gynecologist in the Parke-Davis department of research and development, and told him that I wanted to do a clinical trial on a drug

*The drug is known as Ponstan in Canada and Europe.

called Ponstel, which I felt would be excellent for treating menstrual cramps.

I'm not sure what Dr. Petrick thought that day. I suppose if I had been from the Harvard Medical School department of research he would have been impressed, but I could only say that I was a family doctor hoping to find relief for menstrual pain. Most likely he wondered why he was on the telephone with some crazy lady doctor from Long Island who wanted to get rid of cramps. Anyway, initially Dr. Petrick was somewhat less than enthusiastic. He said, "It's like trying to cure the common cold; we really don't know the mechanism. I'll have to see."

After two days, I felt he had had enough time to "see." I called him back. This time I made sure he understood that all I wanted was some of the drug and their okay to use it. No, I wasn't asking for any money! Just a few bottles of Ponstel, please. I must have gotten my point across, because the drug appeared in the mail that month. I now had a free supply of the drug for my patients and for myself.

I began my study by asking some patients who had been on narcotic medication for their dysmenorrhea to try Ponstel. As the months went on, the women seemed to receive good pain relief, so I gave the drug to more and more women. In a very simple trial, I gave each patient some yellow-and-blue capsules of Ponstel and told her to let me know if it helped and how it compared to other medication she had taken. At the end of five months, thirty-four women had taken the drug and most reported good results. I in turn reported to Parke-Davis that my experiment had been successful. I think they were somewhat surprised at just how effective the drug seemed to be. We decided that the study was worth publishing, if only as a letter to the editor. And so the results of the trial were tabulated and appeared in the *American Journal of Obstetrics and Gynecology* on September 15, 1977.

My small and uncontrolled study showed that 85 percent of the women felt that they got good relief from pain with

Ponstel. Of the sixteen women who used Ponstel for three or more periods, fourteen experienced improvement and ten reported complete relief. Virtually all the women considered Ponstel more effective than aspirin, and most considered Ponstel more effective than Darvon. Eleven women needed no more than three tablets (750 mg) per period to control symptoms. An additional sixteen needed only five to ten capsules, and no woman needed more than sixteen. The doses, well within the approved dosage rate for Ponstel, were tolerated well.[12]

On February 1, 1977, before my small note appeared in the literature, I did what was probably the first television program in the world devoted to menstrual pain. I was in Seattle, Washington, at the time and appeared on "Seattle Today," a live morning TV talk show. Scheduled to speak on a topic concerning women's health, I chose dysmenorrhea because I wanted to give women a better understanding of why they had pain. It took a lot of talking, though, before I finally managed to convince the male producer of the show to let me devote the half-hour to that subject.

The Seattle women watching that show were the first to hear that menstrual pain was not in their heads but was caused by substances called prostaglandins. I had published nothing at the time, and though I told the audience that there was hope of treatment, I did not feel free to tell them the name of the drug I was working with. It was a prescription item, and no doctor would prescribe it without data to back him up. So the main message on that show had to be that menstrual pain is real, and that those who suffer pain should no longer feel guilty or be made to feel guilty.

While I was still on the air, the phones in the studio started ringing and rang continuously for days. That was the biggest response "Seattle Today" had ever received. The overwhelming interest in this women's health matter was entirely unexpected by the station, but I was not surprised. I knew there were a lot of women out there for whom my words were the promise of release from a constantly recurring prison of pain—and guilt. The reality of menstrual problems had been kept under wraps long enough. It was time to bring the subject into the public eye and make the problem visible. Everyone needed to know that menstrual pain was as real as angina—doctors, bosses, and other women, too. And that there *was* relief, safe relief. The media was the best way I knew to get the message across.

The TV station did not give out my address, but letters from viewers found me anyway, rerouted from the medical school where I taught, which had been mentioned on the air. I answered them all, but I gave special attention to the ones from women who said they already had scheduled hysterectomies because they could no longer put up with severe menstrual pain. That jarred me. I couldn't believe that a woman would consider hysterectomy just because of pain; but if so many were saying the same thing, it had to be true. I was horrified. I wrote those women back as quickly as I could, giving them the name of the drug and instructions for taking it. If their physicians would prescribe it, it was likely to work. After all, the drug had been on the market since 1967 for pain. Certainly menstrual pain fits into that general category. If their physicians would co-operate, perhaps these women could be spared a major surgical procedure.

The tremendous response of the Seattle women persuaded me that I had to set up a definitive study to prove that the drug was effective. As Parke-Davis became aware that the drug might be useful to millions of women, the financial reward of undertaking such a study became apparent to them. No longer would I have to support the research. Study patients' office visits and lab work would be paid for by Parke-Davis.

And so a rigidly controlled, scientific, double-blind, cross-over study was set up.

A double-blind study is one in which neither the investigator (me) nor the patient knows whether she is receiving medication or sugar-filled capsules. Crossover means that for half of the experiment, in this case three months, the

patient is on the drug (Ponstel) and then crosses over to
a placebo for the second three months, or vice versa. This
procedure is important, for it prevents the doctor from being
able to influence the outcome of the study. For example,
I might say, "This medication is great, take it and you will
be rid of all your menstrual pain." This could be enough
to influence some patients and slant the study results. Even
the capsules were made up specially for the study: the placebos and the active drug looked identical. Both were an
unappealing brown, because market research has shown that
some people react to the color of pills. Pink, yellow, and
some other pretty pills make you feel better, but all my
capsules were brown precisely because we didn't want to
influence anyone psychologically.

  I had to find fifty women with menstrual cramps to participate in this new study. Since I have a somewhat limited
practice, finding fifty patients with monthly menstrual pain
was a challenge, especially as I needed them quickly. Luckily,
the producer of a weekly Long Island radio show for women
heard of my work on menstrual pain and asked me to do
a program with her. It was the perfect opportunity to tell
a New York audience about the cause of menstrual pain
and to announce that I intended to start a study of a new
treatment for dysmenorrhea. For women who entered the
study, medical care would be free for the next six months.
I told them that the drug to be used was not new or experimental, and it was neither a narcotic nor a hormone.
I got my fifty patients.

  In fact, I got twice that many but selected only those
whose answers to a questionnaire confirmed that they had
spasmodic dysmenorrhea and not congestive dysmenorrhea.
Congestive dysmenorrhea is defined as abdominal discomfort
before the onset of menses, accompanied by bloating, breast
tenderness, and premenstrual tension. Women with congestive dysmenorrhea may have cramps, but their major complaints occur before the menses, and very often the onset
of flow brings relief. Spasmodic dysmenorrhea—the complaint I wanted to work with—is defined as cramping pain

in the lower abdomen that begins at or near the beginning of the monthly flow. Current scientific thinking was that the cramping occurred with the flow due to release of prostaglandins from the menstrual fluid. My study would begin medication with a prostaglandin-inhibiting drug with the onset of flow, so those women with symptoms occurring primarily before the onset of flow would get little benefit from participation.

To distinguish between women with spasmodic dysmenorrhea and those with congestive dysmenorrhea, I administered the questionnaire reprinted on pages 54–55.[13] It asks 25 questions, and each answer can be scored to determine whether your problem occurs *before* menstruation or *during* it and whether your problem is predominately congestive or spasmodic. None of us has only one type of menstrual complaint. All of us have breast tenderness or abdominal crampy discomfort from time to time. Furthermore, one menstrual period is not necessarily like the next. (Men don't know about that yet.) This questionnaire, however, gave an overall indication of whether the complaint was mostly congestive or mostly spasmodic.

Circle the answer that best describes your own typical menstrual cycles. Then score the sheet by separately adding the total spasmodic scores and the total congestive scores, and see which is greater. The higher score indicates your type of monthly problem. Even, or near even scores mean you have a mixture of symptoms. Higher total scores indicate more frequent complaints than lower scores.

When the women had been selected, I decided that we should all get together in my home to discuss the project we were about to embark on. Not many scientific studies are run out of small, private offices, and I felt it was essential that they understand completely their role in the study and that they were free to drop out at any time.

The gatherings turned out to be very heartening. For the first time, each of us had a chance to relate her experiences with menstrual pain to other understanding human beings.

Item*	Never Rarely Sometimes Often Always (1 2 3 4 5)	Type of dysmenorrhea: S = Spasmodic C = Congestive
1. I feel irritable, easily agitated, and am impatient a few days *before* my period.	N R S O A	(C)
2. I have cramps that *begin* on the first day of my period.	N R S O A	(S)
3. I feel depressed for several days *before* my period.	N R S O A	(C)
4. I have abdominal pain or discomfort which begins one day *before* my period.	N R S O A	(S)
5. For several days *before* my period I feel exhausted, lethargic or tired.	N R S O A	(C)
6. I only know that my period is coming by looking at the calendar.	N R S O A	(S)
7. I take a prescription drug for the pain *during* my period.	N R S O A	(S)
8. I feel weak and dizzy *during* my period.	N R S O A	(S)
9. I feel tense and nervous *before* my period.	N R S O A	(C)
10. I have diarrhea *during* my period.	N R S O A	(S)
11. I have backaches several days *before* my period.	N R S O A	(C)
12. I take aspirin for the pain *during* my period.	N R S O A	(S)
13. My breasts feel tender and sore a few days *before* my period.	N R S O A	(C)
14. My lower back, abdomen, and the inner sides of my thighs *begin* to hurt or be tender on the first day of my period.	N R S O A	(S)
15. *During* the first day or so of my period, I feel like curling up in bed, using a hot water bottle on my abdomen, or taking a hot bath.	N R S O A	(S)
16. I gain weight *before* my period.	N R S O A	(C)
17. I am constipated *during* my period.	N R S O A	(C)
18. *Beginning* on the first day of my period, I have pains which may diminish or disappear for several minutes and then reappear.	N R S O A	(S)

*On the first 24 items patients were instructed to indicate the degree to which they experience the symptom by selecting one of five response choices [Never (N), Rarely (R), Sometimes (S), Often (O), and Always (A)].

Item	Never Rarely Sometimes Often Always (1 2 3 4 5)	Type of dysmenorrhea: S = Spasmodic C = Congestive
19. The pain I have with my period is not intense, but a continuous dull aching.	N R S O A	(C)
20. I have abdominal discomfort for more than one day *before* my period.	N R S O A	(C)
21. I have backaches which *begin* the same day as my period.	N R S O A	(S)
22. My abdominal area feels bloated for a few days *before* my period.	N R S O A	(C)
23. I feel nauseated *during* the first day or so of my period.	N R S O A	(S)
24. I have headaches for a few days *before* my period.	N R S O A	(C)
25. TYPE 1 or TYPE 2*		

*On the twenty-fifth item, patients were instructed to read the descriptions of two types of menstrual discomfort and select the type that most closely fits their experience. If Type 1, add 5 to spasmodic score. If Type 2, add 5 to congestive score.

TYPE 1

The pain begins on the first day of menstruation, often coming within an hour of the first signs of menstruation. The pain is most severe the first day and may or may not continue on subsequent days. Felt as spasms, the pain may lessen or subside for awhile and then reappear. A few women find this pain so severe as to cause vomiting, fainting or dizziness; some others report that they are most comfortable in bed or taking a hot bath. This pain is limited to the lower abdomen, back and inner sides of the thighs.

TYPE 2

There is advance warning of the onset of menstruation during which the woman feels an increasing heaviness, and a dull aching in the lower abdomen. This pain is sometimes accompanied by nausea, lack of appetite, and constipation. Headaches, backaches, and breast pain are also characteristic of this type of menstrual discomfort.

The type that most closely fits my experience is TYPE _____.

A 41-year-old woman with five children stated that her menstrual cramps were still terrible. She was using an IUD for birth control. I had to tell her that there could be no women in the study who were on the pill, had IUDs, or had pelvic abnormalities, because these factors affect menstrual cycles and pain and would confuse the study results. After the others had left, she said, "Please, take out my IUD. I want to be in your study." I did.

One of the women, a concert pianist, wanted to have a hysterectomy rather than face more menstrual pain. Hysterectomy, to her, seemed like a pleasant alternative. My study was her last hope.

One woman told us that when she was expecting her first baby, people told her she could judge when she was supposed to leave for the hospital by the fact that her labor contractions would become as hard and as painful as her menstrual cramps. She said, laughingly, that she almost gave birth in her living room because her labor pains never reached the point where they were half as painful as her cramps.

Another woman chimed in to say that she had had exactly the same experience. She had four children, and every labor was easier than her monthly menstrual pain. She wanted to join the study because, with four children and a busy social life, she couldn't afford twenty-four days out of each year in bed. As she put it, "That's almost a month out of my life every year." One or two women were unable to come to the gatherings because they were incapacitated by menstrual pain. The most common comment at each gathering was that you could always count on having your menstrual pain whenever you were doing something important, like taking college exams or having job interviews or auditions.

There were three such get-togethers. I wanted to talk individually to all fifty of the participants and take the time to answer all their questions. My most important recollection from the meetings was how dedicated the women were. They really wanted to free women from menstrual pain. Some of my missionary fervor had evidently rubbed off.

Since I met my criteria for inclusion, I became one of the research subjects, too. I have always felt that I would not ask a patient to participate in any study in which I myself would not. Taking my own Pap smear proved a little tricky, but other than that, I had no problem being both researcher and subject.

We were told to begin taking the capsules containing placebo or active drug at the onset of flow and to take four daily for a maximum of three days. We could take less if our pain decreased. No one was allowed to use aspirin, aspirin-containing products, or Tylenol. If the medication did not give pain relief, the only additional drug allowed was a half-grain of codeine. The rules were strictly enforced.

Patients had to return after each period and fill out a form. They also had to tell me how that month had been in comparison to their usual cycles. After I had asked them their usual questions, they would often inquire how I was doing.

I was positive that I had the "good stuff" during my first three months, because my cramps didn't exist. I had to tell several of the patients who were not getting relief to hang in there because better days would be coming. I modified that statement every time with, "Of course, it's possible that the drug might not work for you."

Four women dropped out of the study. One unexpectedly became pregnant after twelve years of marriage and infertility, one could not make long trips into the office on a monthly basis, and two couldn't put up with what turned out to be placebos and codeine for three months. I can't say that I blame them. If I had gotten placebo first and had had pain for three months, with or without codeine, I wouldn't have been too happy, either.

Each month, a research assistant from Parke-Davis came to my office to pick up the patient data. I completed the data as soon as possible, hoping to expedite the preliminary work that had to be done for the computer runs. All the patients finished in December 1977, and the data were in. A few weeks later, the code that told who was on which drug was shown to us. It seemed to me that most of the women in the study had been right about which capsule was effective and which was not.

Computer time was at a premium. Parke-Davis had other projects that were considered more important than menstrual-cramp studies to run on their computers. I waited for almost a year. Finally the data were ready in late 1978, and I prepared the final draft of my report.

The next question was where to publish the results. I did not want to publish the study in a journal for gynecologists only, because family doctors, internists, and pediatricians were often confronted with the menstrual-cramp problem. Instead, I selected the *Journal of the American Medical Association (JAMA),* because it reaches the widest range and greatest number of doctors; and the *Journal* agreed to print the article. After six months, in late May of 1979, I called *JAMA* and asked when the article would appear. The woman on the other end of the line replied after checking, "Well, everything is in order. It will be published when it is picked."

I responded, "You mean, it's just sitting there waiting to be 'picked' while millions of women are suffering each month?"

Silence.

"You publish articles every week on diseases so exotic and rare that only four cases have ever been noted in the literature. Dysmenorrhea doesn't kill anyone, but it certainly makes life miserable for millions of women. The number of women who have this problem makes it important to publish this article now."

I never knew if my phone call did any good, but the article was published at the end of the next month, June 22, 1979, as the lead article. It reported:

Dysmenorrhea is a frequent complaint that lacks safe, specific therapy. Narcotics are often prescribed that give some relief but make it difficult for women to function effectively, or birth control pills may be administered for twenty-one days to afford twenty-four hours' relief of pain.

Recent evidence indicates that endometrial prostaglandins of the E and F series cause the painful uterine contractions and the systemic signs of primary spasmodic dysmenorrhea. . . . The discovery that nonsteroidal anti-inflammatory agents inhibit prostaglandin synthesis provides a rationale for the use of these agents in the treatment of primary spasmodic dysmenorrhea.

Mefenamic acid (Ponstel), introduced in 1967, is the only fenamate analgesic available in this country. The fenamate compounds have been shown to act as inhibitors of both prostaglandin synthesis and prostaglandin activity.

To sum up the results of the study, Ponstel produced

highly significant relief in frequency and severity of the symptoms in forty-four women with primary spasmodic dysmenorrhea.

Pain relief and drug benefit were somewhat greater among patients who received mefenamic acid after crossing over from placebo than among those who received it before placebo. . . . It may be that transfer from placebo to mefenamic acid induced relatively more relief because the patient had been without effective treatment for the three preceding cycles.

The patients required much less or no codeine while on Ponstel than on placebo. Also, they felt significantly greater relief from nausea-vomiting and weakness-dizziness while they were on Ponstel. Patients also commented on two other effects: leg achiness diminished, and menstrual flow decreased.

Adverse reactions were infrequent during the study. In fact, more patients reported stomach upsets while on placebo (five) than while on Ponstel (three). There were no significant changes in blood or urine values.[14]

The fact that the drug proved effective in a rigid double-blind study was especially significant. An average of 85 percent of the women were relieved of their pain. The statistics were even better than I had dared hope. A double-blind study with such excellent results carries a lot of weight. To me, it had special meaning, for not only did it prove that the drug worked extremely well, but it also proved that placebo was essentially worthless. Women with dysmen-

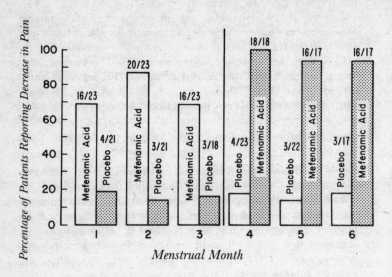

orrhea have physical pain that will not respond to placebo
or psychological suggestion. Dysmenorrhea is a physiologic
problem that needs specific therapy.

The psychological theory of menstrual pain was dead.

The research effort was over. The study had been published, but I felt that my work was not yet finished. I had
often lectured about how important it is for doctors to keep
abreast of developments in medicine, and that it is equally
important for women to be educated on new developments
in women's health. I had even delivered a paper on just
that subject at the International Medical Women's Association meeting in August 1978 in Berlin.

Thus I was upset when it turned out that even experts
in the field of women's-health literature for physicians didn't
seem to appreciate the major breakthrough that had occurred
in the treatment of dysmenorrhea. A well-written article on
dysmenorrhea was buried in one of the women's health care
professional journals, its presence not even noted on the

cover of the magazine. I called the assistant editor of the journal and said, "Dr. Dawood wrote an excellent article. Why didn't you feature it on the front of the journal? You headlined other articles that aren't nearly as important as his."

"You're right," she said, as though it were an adequate explanation. "We goofed."

If even the literature of the medical profession neglected the good news about dysmenorrhea treatment, how could I possibly spread the word? It didn't take me long to think of a way. I had often watched a Sunday morning television program devoted to new research developments in medicine, which was hosted by Frank Field, a New York health commentator on NBC television. It occurred to me that he might be interested in reporting on dysmenorrhea and how aspirin and the newer antiprostaglandin medicine worked. I remember looking up at my office nurse and asking, "Do you think Frank Field might be interested?" I never waited for her puzzled look to clear, but dialed the phone.

Frank Field was interested all right. He said, "I'm so glad you called. I was going to call you today. I read your study in *JAMA* and I think it's very exciting. I'd like to come out to your laboratories and film a story—tomorrow. I want your research on the Sunday news."

I wasn't quite prepared for this; my head was still thinking about his intellectual Sunday morning medical research program that dealt in depth with new medical discoveries and therapies. I explained that all I had was an office, a small one at that, but he was welcome.

Suddenly he said, "This is really very important news for women. You have to be on the 'Today' show, on Monday!"

"No, no, not Monday morning, I have office hours."

"Okay, Tuesday."

Early the next morning, Frank Field arrived at my office with a camera crew. We chatted for about fifteen minutes so that he would understand the research and know what questions to ask. We filmed for about ten minutes. He suggested that he would also like to interview a couple of patients who had taken the drug, so I phoned two patients who lived nearby. From those interviews, he edited the most important parts to put on the air.

The interview was broadcast on Sunday night. First thing Monday morning, I received a call from Frank Field.

"If it's possible, I'd like to interview you on tonight's six o'clock news. The phones were ringing like crazy last night after the news."

So I finished my office hours a little early and drove into Manhattan. I took clothes with me for the next morning, too, because on Tuesday I had to be in the city at 7 A.M. for the "Today" show.

After I arrived at the studio and I sat down to have my face powdered, a young woman thrust her hand at me.

"I'm Frank Field's assistant. I think I have dysmenorrhea of the ear. I answered more than three hundred calls about your research yesterday."

As bad as it had seemed to her, it got worse. After the "Today" show, NBC switchboards were overloaded for the entire day and most of the next. My appearances prompted more phone calls to NBC than they had ever received before. Many women had heard for the first time that they were not "head cases" because they suffered from menstrual pain. They also heard that a drug was available to end their monthly woes. Neither I nor Frank Field had ever envisioned the splash that all of this would make.

One New York City reporter, however, wasn't pleased with this media coverage. He complained that the drug had not been approved for menstrual pain, and that I should not be talking about its use for that purpose. To be truthful, I hadn't been concerned about that nicety. The drug had been on the market since 1967 for pain relief. Menstrual pain was pain. It was a moot point to me that the drug company had no Food and Drug Administration (FDA) okay to advertise Ponstel for that specific type of pain. I felt that too many women had waited too long already. Any doctor who wanted to prescribe it could do so legitimately because he was treating pain.

Dr. Petrick from Parke-Davis called me, too. "Wow," he said, "I think it's great to have such interest, but it's possible the FDA will be unhappy about your publicity. They haven't given us approval to advertise for menstrual-pain relief yet— and they may not."

However, the story had caught the fancy of too many others, and containment was no longer possible.

I almost didn't make it through the next six weeks. My office hours ran one to two hours behind because the phones were always ringing with calls from almost all the major women's magazines and radio and television stations. There were also many phone calls from women who wanted information about the drug. Doctors began requesting reprints of the *JAMA* article.

For those six weeks, I ran a menstrual questionnaire office. Finally I got smart and put a form letter together to send to women who wanted drug information. In it, I attempted to answer their questions about antiprostaglandin drugs and other drug regimens used in the past and still used by physicians to attempt to alleviate the symptoms of severe dysmenorrhea.

For example, frequently narcotics such as codeine or oxycodone (Percodan) are used to combat the pain, and they can be effective. However, the patient is, in general, unable to function. Sometimes, when pain is particularly severe, narcotics are ineffective, and some women, though they are in a semistuporous state, may still suffer menstrual pain for one to three days each month. One of my patients described this condition as having her head swimming and sleepy, but her cramps still hurting. The possibility of addiction must also be kept in mind with narcotics, particularly when they are taken in increasingly higher dosages over extended periods of time.

Oral contraceptives (the pill) have also been used with considerable success to treat menstrual pain. Their synthetic hormones prevent ovulation and also tend to thin the uterine lining, thereby decreasing prostaglandin production and the problems of dysmenorrhea. From a logical medical stand-point, however, this treatment should be considered only by those women who wish to use these medications primarily for birth control, with a secondary benefit of dysmenorrhea relief. They are taken daily for three weeks out of every four, and to expose one's body to constant hormonal therapy in order to obtain relief from menstrual pain for only twenty-four to thirty-six hours of each month is absurd in my judg-ment, unless it is also the patient's choice for contraception.

Some other drugs used are antispasmodics, which relax the gastrointestinal tract and stop its overactivity. Doctors assume that they will also relieve uterine overactivity; but my experience tells me that antispasmodic drugs simply don't work well on dysmenorrhea.

Sadly, the minor tranquilizers also have been used by some physicians, apparently to relieve emotional stress that is per-ceived to be causing the menstrual pain. And many women have resorted to psychiatry after having been convinced by their physicians and others that their monthly physical dis-ability is largely a manifestation of emotional disorders.

Unfortunately, diet (including extra calcium), exercise, psy-chiatric intervention, and relaxation do not seem to be any more helpful than placebos.

I also tell my patients about the many nonprescription remedies for menstrual pain that are available at drugstores. Some of these preparations, which have been around for decades, probably provide some relief to women who suffer from mild dysmenorrhea. Many of them contain aspirin or aspirin derivatives. I am convinced that aspirin, taken by itself, is probably as good as and perhaps superior to most of these remedies since it is a mild antiprostaglandin. In addition to aspirin, these over-the-counter preparations gen-erally contain antihistamines for sedation and antispasmodics such as cinnamedrine and homatropine. These ingredients usually are present in less than effective doses. Several prep-arations contain caffeine to provide a stimulant effect.

Some Nonprescription Remedies for Dysmenorrhea

Brand	Ingredients
Femcaps Capsules (Buffington)	aspirin 2.5 gr, phenacetin 1 gr, caffeine citrate 0.5 gr, ephedrine sulfate 0.06 mg, atropine sulfate 0.03 mg
Femicin (Norcliff-Thayer)	salicylamide 225 mg, acetaminophen 160 mg, caffeine 65 mg, pyrilamine maleate 15 mg, homatropine MBr 0.5 mg
Her-Caps (EJ Moore)	acetaminophen 120 mg, salicylamide 210 mg, caffeine 30 mg, calcium gluconate 60 mg
Mense (Rbt. Daniels)	aspirin 227 mg, acetaminophen 65 mg, phenacetin 162 mg, caffeine 32.4 mg
Midol (Glenbrook)	aspirin 454 mg, caffeine 32.4 mg, cinnamedrine 14.9 mg

WITH DIURETIC

Brand	Ingredients
Aqua-Ban (Thompson Medical)	ammonium chloride 325 mg, caffeine 100 mg
Cadui (Chattem)	salicylamide 250 mg, phenacetin 125 mg, pamabrom 25 mg, pyrilamine maleate 12.5 mg
Femeze (Stanlabs)	acetaminophen, salicylamide, caffeine, ammonium chloride, vitamin B_1, homatropine MBr
Flowaway Water (DeWitt)	uva ursi extract 98 mg, buchu leaves extract 24 mg, caffeine 20 mg, potassium nitrate 171 mg
Fluidex (O'Connor)	buchu powdered extract 65 mg, couch grass powdered extract 65 mg, cornsilk powdered extract 32.5 mg, hydrangea powdered extract 32.5 mg
Fluidex-Plus with Diadax (O'Connor)	above plus phenylpropanolamine Hcl 25 mg
Odrinil (Fox)	powdered extract of buchu 34.4 mg, uva ursi 34.4 mg, cornsilk 34.4 mg, juniper 16.2 mg, caffeine extract 16.2 mg

Some Nonprescription Remedies for Dysmenorrhea

WITH DIURETIC

Pamprin (Chattem)	acetaminophen 325 mg, pamabrom 25 mg, pyrilamine maleate 12.5 mg
Pre-Mens Forte (Blair)	ammonium chloride 500 mg, caffeine 100 mg
Sunril (Schering)	acetaminophen 300 mg, pamabrom 50 mg, pyrilamine maleate 25 mg
Trendar (Whitehall)	acetaminophen 325 mg, pamabrom 25 mg, phenindamine tartrate 12.5 mg

OTHER

Humphrey's No. 11 (Humphrey's Pharmacal)	cimicifuga, pulsatilla, sepia
Lydia Pinkham (Smith Miller Patch)	extract of Jamaica dogwood, pleurisy root, and licorice; ferrous sulfate
Lydia Pinkham Vegetable Compound Liquid (Smith Miller Patch)	extract of Jamaica dogwood, pleurisy root, and licorice; alcohol

Finally I tell my patients about antiprostaglandins, starting with the simplest of them, which is aspirin. Introduced in tablet form in 1915, aspirin is consumed by Americans at the rate of over twelve thousand tons a year, the equivalent of more than 150 tablets per person.[15] It is little wonder that we tend to forget that aspirin is a drug, but aspirin is so potent that if it were submitted today to the FDA for approval, it would almost certainly be classified as a prescription item, not to be sold over the counter.

Aspirin has three major effects: it reduces fever, it reduces pain, and it reduces inflammation. Aspirin and other closely related nonsteroidal, anti-inflammatory drugs are also known to be effective in reducing the prostaglandin-induced contraction of smooth muscle. Absorbed from the stomach and upper small intestine and rapidly distributed throughout the body, aspirin works by interfering with the manufacture of prostaglandin in the temperature-regulatory center located in the brain. It reduces pain by blocking prostaglandin synthesis at the site of the pain. And it reduces inflammation by inhibiting synthesis of the prostaglandins that create it. Aspirin, however, is only partially effective as an inhibitor of the synthesis of prostaglandins. Other related compounds—such as Ponstel; Motrin, produced by Upjohn; Anaprox, produced by Syntex; Zomax, produced by McNeil; and Indocin, manufactured by Merck, Sharpe & Dohme—are much more effective in this activity. Indocin, an older antiprostaglandin currently used by some doctors for the treatment of dysmenorrhea, frequently has side effects (including stomach ulceration, bleeding, and perforation; and headache) and should be used only if Motrin, Ponstel, and Anaprox have been tried and found to be ineffective.

There are side effects common to the whole group of antiprostaglandins. The more usual symptoms include indigestion, heartburn, nausea, vomiting, and diarrhea. Most of these gastrointestinal side effects can be prevented simply by taking the medication with milk or food, but because gastrointestinal problems are common during dysmenorrhea, it is often hard to tell whether symptoms should be attributed to the drug or the dysmenorrhea itself. In addition, most of the more serious known side effects of antiprostaglandins, such as anemia, have occurred after six to eighteen months of continuous daily use in therapy for chronic, long-term illness, primarily arthritis. It would seem logical that such side effects would be less when the drugs are given for dysmenorrhea only one or two days each month.

Reasons to avoid taking antiprostaglandins include:

1. Aspirin-induced asthma. If aspirin causes you to have an asthmatic attack, you should not use any of these compounds, because they are all closely related to aspirin and may cause the same reaction. The same advice follows if you get hives or nasal polyps from aspirin.
2. Chronic inflammation or ulceration of the upper or lower gastrointestinal tract.
3. Age limitations. Ponstel should not be given to children

under 14 years of age, since safe use in this age group
has not been established in the United States. (However,
Ponstel is used widely in Africa for infants and children.
It is known there as the "fever reliever.") Motrin has
a lower age limit of 12 years. Anaprox is not recommended for children for the same reasons. (Syntex con-
siders menstruating females no longer children for
prescribing purposes.)

4. Sensitivity to the drug.

Should rash or diarrhea occur, the drug should be stopped.
Ponstel should not be administered for more than a week,
but the other drugs have no such limitation. None of these
drugs should be taken with aspirin. Codeine or acetamin-
ophen, on the other hand, could be taken if necessary. It
would make more sense to try another antiprostaglandin,
however, rather than a narcotic if the particular antiprostaglandin medication you are taking is not giving you good
pain relief. Each of us has her own particular body chemistry,
and you may find that one antiprostaglandin drug works
much better than another for you.

Ponstel has been on the market in the United States for
mild to moderate pain since 1967. In August 1979 Parke-
Davis began advertising Ponstel for menstrual-pain relief.
The menstrual-pain promotion was withdrawn, however,
while the FDA accumulated information on long-term use.
The FDA has now officially approved Ponstel for alleviation
of menstrual pain.

Motrin, another anti-inflammatory drug produced by Upjohn, also has been approved for treatment of mild to moderate pain including menstrual pain. (Upjohn has been a
world leader in prostaglandin study and has funded much
of the European and American research.) After Motrin had
been approved in September 1974 for use against the pain
of arthritis, Upjohn looked for other types of pain that might
be treated by the drug. In 1976, unknown to me, they ini-
tiated dental and dysmenorrhea studies. Researchers proved
that Motrin relieved pain, reduced uterine activity, reduced

intrauterine pressure, and decreased prostaglandin levels in the menstrual fluid. These studies led to the approval of the use of Motrin for the pain of dysmenorrhea.

Similar clinical and technical studies have demonstrated the usefulness of Anaprox for dysmenorrhea. It has received FDA approval also.

During this same time period, research began in England[16] and Europe.[17] All research led to the same conclusion: antiprostaglandin medication was extremely effective in combating the pain of dysmenorrhea.

Studies are under way to compare one drug's effectiveness to the other, but it seems to me that the drugs are approximately equally effective. They all stop the manufacture of prostaglandins, thereby removing the substance that is causing the muscle spasms and the resultant pain. Getting rid of the excessive amounts of prostaglandins also quiets the gut and blood-vessel activity. This in turn stops the nausea, vomiting, diarrhea, and flushes. These drugs do not abolish the contractions completely but bring them down to normal levels.

I give my patients precise instructions for taking antiprostaglandins. This is very important. They must be taken correctly to get the best result. Menstrual cramps usually begin either with the onset of flow or within two to three hours. A couple of capsules should be carried with you so they are available when the period begins.

One or two capsules, depending on the initial degree of pain you experience, should be taken with milk at the very first sign of spotting. After that, you can take one capsule every four to six hours as needed. Only as many capsules as are required should be taken. The maximum dose in United States prescribing literature is five capsules per day, but I often tell my patients that they may take six per day (the usual dose prescribed in Europe). Most women only need the medication for one to two days, and many take only two to four capsules per month. Others, with severe problems or during especially bad months, may take up to twenty-five capsules per month.

If you have cramps that begin on the second day of your flow, then you may start your medication that second day. If that does not work out as well as you would like, take two to four capsules the first day (after meals, with milk), and then take what you need (up to six) the second day.

Women who have pain one to two days before the onset of their periods can begin taking the medication with the onset of their cramps. This should not be done, however, if there is any possibility that you might be pregnant, because pregnant women may get cramps from time to time and not realize that they are pregnant. I want to emphasize that pregnant women should not be exposed to any drugs, and that includes alcohol, caffeine, and cigarettes.

The directions for Motrin are similar. Take the first pill at the first sign of spotting or pain and repeat every four to six hours until there is good pain relief. The maximum dosage for 400-milligram Motrin tablets is six per day also.

For Anaprox, the directions are to take two tablets immediately, followed by one tablet every six to eight hours as needed. The total daily dose should not exceed five tablets.

If none of the antiprostaglandins works, it could mean that you have dysmenorrhea that is not caused by prostaglandins, or, more likely, that you have a pelvic problem that has not been properly diagnosed. You should see your doctor again.

The search for even more specific drugs goes on—drugs that will give quicker relief, act only on the uterine prostaglandins, have fewer side effects, and, one day soon, need no prescription. Researchers are now being flooded with requests from drug manufacturers to investigate new antiprostaglandin drugs for possible use against dysmenorrhea.

Some people look upon the drug companies' sudden interest in dysmenorrhea as only another greedy bid to make money in a newly discovered market. But I welcome it and will be part of the continuing research effort, studying promising new drugs. I am completing a research study on another promising drug called Zomax. Preliminary data would seem

to indicate that Zomax will soon be added to the arma-
mentarium for dysmenorrhea. The more effective drugs we
can find, the better; because if one medication doesn't work
well for some women, another may. Furthermore, should
you become mildly allergic to one, you can simply switch
to another, unless you have asthma or an equally serious
difficulty that is caused by the drug.

So whatever the underlying reason for the newfound interest in dysmenorrhea, it is certainly long overdue and
should result in making life better for women. The more
research, and the more researchers involved, the more facts
will be uncovered about this age-old problem, until finally
the day will come when there will be "no more menstrual
cramps."

CHAPTER 2

No More Premenstrual Syndrome

For many women, the pain of dysmenorrhea is only part of their menstrual difficulties. Many also suffer from a whole complex of symptoms known as premenstrual syndrome. Although the timing of the symptoms varies from one woman to the next, a particular woman will usually experience her symptoms at the same point in her cycle. And no matter when she gets them—whether mid-cycle or immediately before menstruation—the package of symptoms is known as premenstrual syndrome.

I doubt that any woman is unfortunate enough to experience the whole catastrophe, but almost every woman usually suffers one or more of the symptoms, and the cluster is almost always the same for each woman. The symptoms can be classified in the following manner:

psychological: irritability, lethargy, depression, anxiety, sleep disorders, crying spells, hostility
neurological: headache (migraines usually occur the week preceding menstruation), dizziness, fainting, or, rarely, seizures
glandular: tenderness and swelling of breasts

gastrointestinal: constipation, abdominal bloating, abdominal
  cramping, craving for sweets
urinary: less frequent urination
dermatological: acne on face

Women note the appearance of their symptoms by saying
that they feel out of sorts or "witchy"; but no matter what
name they give it, every woman recognizes the event. Unfortunately, she may not recognize that she is experiencing
premenstrual syndrome until she actually begins to flow,
while a husband or lover may note the onset of the symptoms,
assure himself that it is just "that time of the month," and
try to keep a low profile. As Robert Kinch observed:

> Often a patient will tell you she fails to associate her behavior
> with menstruation until the period actually begins. But the hus-
> band usually does recognize the link and the patient may resent
> his pointing out the connection. . . . This is mother's bad week,
> try not to upset her. . . . In my experience, during the premen-
> strual period, most patients with this syndrome have savage feel-
> ings about everything and are experiencing both self-dislike and
> remorse about their behavior. They tend to withdraw from con-
> tact with other people so as not to make matters worse.[1]

The most common psychological symptom of premenstrual
syndrome is tension; in fact, many people still refer to the
whole syndrome as premenstrual tension. There are three
types of tension: depression, irritability, or lethargy. A sudden mood swing often heralds their arrival.

For some working women, lethargy is the most troublesome symptom; it can have a serious impact on a woman's
career. She may be unable to work at an acceptable pace.
And since lethargy is extremely difficult to overcome, she
may want nothing more than to sneak back to bed and stay
there.

The depression that often occurs with premenstrual syndrome, however, can be the most serious symptom of all. The woman who is affected with this symptom weeps easily and is generally on a super "downer." She feels totally inadequate and convinced that no one really cares about her. She thinks she lacks the concentration to make decisions or take examinations. She is upset by almost anything. Even though the depression lasts for only a few days, it can be very severe.

Some women abuse alcohol during this premenstrual time. In a survey of menstruating female alcoholics, 67 percent of the women related the start of a drinking bout with that time in their menstrual cycle.[2] An interesting study done at the University of Oklahoma gave female study subjects 0.3 milliliters of alcohol per pound of body weight. They found that women had the highest blood alcohol levels when they were premenstrual and became more obviously intoxicated during their premenstrual time. Dr. F. Seixas, who wrote a report on the female alcoholic, stated,

> A woman who may not feel high on three drinks taken near the middle of her menstrual cycle when hormone levels are highest may become quite drunk on the same amount of alcohol ingested at the end of her menstrual cycle when hormone levels have dropped.[3]

Many studies of suicide attempts, either successful or unsuccessful, have shown an increased incidence during the premenstrual week. It is doubtful that premenstrual syndrome drives women to suicide, but it is possible that the depression of premenstrual syndrome worsens a preexisting depression and may be enough to trigger a suicide attempt.

Despite the seriousness of these symptoms, premenstrual-syndrome sufferers who seek professional help from physicians to deal with their symptoms have traditionally been treated with a pep talk or a tranquilizer. For generations, premenstrual syndrome, like dysmenorrhea, has been in a medical never-never land. Scant attention has been paid to women who had only minor discomforting symptoms, while women who developed obvious physical symptoms such as swelling or overt severe depression were treated only for these particular complaints. There has been an appalling lack of research on the basic underlying causes of premenstrual syndrome so that specific treatment can be prescribed.

In place of research, we have the widespread, ancient, and firm conviction that no matter what its origins, premenstrual syndrome is dreadfully incapacitating to women. A few years ago, when I was in South Africa lecturing at Groote Schuur Hospital on my research on menstrual pain and the treatment of menopause, I appeared on a television talk show to discuss the fact that South African Airlines did not want female pilots flying their planes because, of course, premenstrual tension supposedly makes women unreliable and unsafe. I was invited to appear on the show not only because of my menstruation research but because I have a private pilot's license. Also on the show was a marvelous American stunt pilot, Grace the Ace, who was performing in South Africa at the time. She and I agreed emphatically that women should be pilots.

"I have my ups and downs," Grace acknowledged, "just like any person—female or male. Believe me, I know plenty of male pilots who have their off days."

"I never have premenstrual tension, but I have slight breast tenderness from month to month," I pursued. "That's no reason to ground a woman."

Yet the attitude of South African Airlines is pretty common all over the world. We all know that women are denied many opportunities because conventional wisdom holds that they will invariably fail to perform at critical times, overcome by their "raging hormones." Medical science has been very conscientious about recording the symptoms of premenstrual syndrome. Psychiatrists and men in general have used such data to justify assigning women a second-class status in society. Corporations have perfected unspoken value systems that equate being female with being emotionally unfit for highly responsible jobs that require "male stability."

But the truth of the matter may be quite different. One

study by **Gamberals, Strindberg, and Wohlberg** and another by Munchell demonstrate that even women who suffer severe menstrual distress do not necessarily suffer any mental impairment or loss of ability to function during their period of distress. Munchell concluded that even though many women function at their normal level during their distress, they falsely believe that they are functioning at a lower level because they have been conditioned to expect that they will. A 1980 study in California showed that women's test scores remained constant at all days in their menstrual cycles.

In other words, while some women probably don't perform up to standard while they are suffering from premenstrual syndrome, many others only think they are not functioning up to par; but in either case, women don't get much assistance from a male-oriented medical establishment that is all too willing to catalog the grim symptoms of being female while doing nothing to relieve them.

Most often, doctors seem content to write off premenstrual syndrome as a psychosomatic illness. Dr. Robert Kinch discussed the psychosomatic causes of premenstrual syndrome in terms that are strikingly similar to many "explanations" of menstrual cramps:

> There is considerable evidence to support a psychic origin of the premenstrual syndrome. Some authorities believe that both the onset and exacerbation of premenstrual tension are precipitated by disturbances that take place in the patient's life.
>
> Patients with this syndrome are thought to have hostile, dependent relationships with their mothers, with subsequent strong feelings of guilt. Or they may repudiate the feminine role and have strong feelings of envy toward men.
>
> I often find that patients with the most difficulties are intelligent women whose abilities and ambitions to explore outside interests are frustrated by child care and other domestic and social responsibilities. Many such patients are married to workaholic professionals.[4]

Sound familiar? It's the same tune that used to be played to explain why women have menstrual pain. But I am convinced that premenstrual syndrome is no more in your head than dysmenorrhea is. I believe that it has an actual chemical basis. As yet, we haven't found the cause—but I'm working on it.

I must admit that I too have been misled by the mythology of premenstrual syndrome. When I spoke about menstrual problems at the International Medical Women's Conference in Berlin in August 1978, I was astonished to receive a great many questions from women doctors from the developing countries of Africa. I still somehow thought that menstrual problems occurred mainly amid the everyday urban stress of developed countries. There I was, supposedly an expert, going around the world to lecture against the myths, and they still had a hold on me. The questions of women from developing countries, however, seemed to confirm Janiger's earlier findings in studies of twenty-four different societies that premenstrual syndrome is not related to the complexity of any given society but is a universal phenomenon. I now believe that if premenstrual tension is in your head, it's probably in your brain chemistry—not in your psyche.

One of the first physicians to become interested in premenstrual syndrome was Dr. Katharina Dalton, who practices in London. In 1953, she published the first paper to appear in the British medical literature on the subject and she has continued to gather data on the impact of premenstrual syndrome on women. Her work made the medical community aware of the seriousness of premenstrual syndrome, in terms of the havoc it causes women and society as a whole; but it is controversial on two counts. First, it seems to confirm that women are unstable, an opinion long used to justify keeping women out of responsible positions. And second, attempts by other researchers to duplicate her experiments and verify her conclusions have failed.

Dalton documented that an unusually high amount of bizarre behavior occurs during the four days before and the four days after the onset of menstruation. She named this

eight-day period—during which some women are more apt
to have accidents, commit crime, or attempt suicide—the
paramenstrum. (It might also be conceivable that a dispro-
portionate number of women in the paramenstrum get married, join a church, or give money to charity, but nobody
has studied those possibilities. Why is it that researchers
always seem to expect the worst of women?)

Dalton's data showed that at four London teaching hospitals, 52 percent of the female admissions due to accidents
occurred during the paramenstrum.[5] The United States Center for Safety Education found that most accidents suffered
by women were likely to occur during the forty-eight hours
before menstruation. Forty-six percent of the acute admissions for psychiatric illness occur during this period. Forty-
nine percent of the newly incarcerated female prisoners in
a women's prison committed their crimes during the paramenstrum. Apparently, then, there is some change in the
emotional stability of the women who experience premenstrual syndrome.

Dalton theorized that premenstrual syndrome occurs as
a result of the precipitous drop in progesterone levels that
occurs at the time of menstruation. She treated hundreds
of women with progesterone and reported very good results
in alleviating the symptoms. But she has not performed a
carefully controlled double-bind study to verify the efficiency
of progesterone in the treatment of premenstrual syndrome.
Meanwhile, other researchers in England have run controlled
studies with progesterone. They have never been able to
duplicate her results.

One of them, Dr. Gwyneth Sampson in Sheffield, England,
attempted to duplicate Dr. Dalton's results, using her methods of giving progesterone and her exact dosage in a controlled double-blind study. She performed a trial on thirty-
nine patients, treated with progesterone and with placebo,
who rated the effect of the treatment they received for each
cycle. These patient ratings suggest " . . . that there is no
difference between progesterone and placebo, and in fact
placebo is always rated more effective, although this is not

significant."[6] Sampson went on to say that whether they received progesterone or placebo, 60 percent of the patients reported being helped by the first treatment cycles—a percentage similar to the success rates claimed for other treatments of premenstrual syndrome. This fact suggests that most women will respond favorably to *any* treatment for premenstrual syndrome, at least for the first cycle.

Although other researchers have not confirmed Dalton's findings, progesterone probably does provide relief for some women. I have used injectable progesterone successfully in a few patients who suffered from severe premenstrual migraine. One study on progesterone given to male volunteers showed brain-wave patterns similar to those obtained using minor tranquilizers such as Valium.[7] After testing several progestogens (synthetic progesterone-like drugs), the researchers concluded that all progestogens have an anxiety-releasing effect on the brain, acting much like tranquilizers do. Other trials with male volunteers reported in recent literature have confirmed this conclusion; and it has in fact become the rationale for treating male sex offenders with progesterone. In these cases, progesterone's tranquilizing effects seem to decrease aggression and violent outbursts. Studies conducted on women being treated for cancer with huge intravenous doses of progesterone noted that they fell asleep within five to fifteen minutes of administration.[8]

Other interesting brain-wave (electroencephalograph or EEG) studies done on women suggest another avenue for research. In the *South African Medical Journal,* Dr. P. M. Leary reported on the results of a study in which he recorded EEGs in twenty-five women at the midpoint of the menstrual cycle and again one day before menstruation. Most premenstrual recordings, in contrast to mid-cycle recordings, showed an increase in brain-wave frequency and amplitude. Leary speculated that the increased brain-wave activity might correspond to mood changes brought on by neurochemical changes in the brain, which were, in turn, modulated by female hormonal shifts. He also suggested that these premenstrual changes might even account for the tendency of certain epileptic women to have seizures only at the time preceding their menses.[9] It would, I think, be of great benefit if this kind of study could be set up in the United States, so that EEG recordings could be compiled for a larger group of women to see if the same results can be obtained. Such a study might also test the efficacy of various medications that seem promising.

Still other investigators of the possible causes of premenstrual syndrome have been studying prolactin, a hormone secreted by the pituitary gland in the brain. Prolactin controls the nursing reflex, which causes milk to flow when the mother's breast is suckled, and it also has a role in controlling the output of ovarian hormones. It is known to be associated with water retention. A high level is found immediately after delivery, when the postpartum blues occur; prolactin levels drop with the start of menstruation, which usually relieves premenstrual syndrome. It is possible that prolactin and the associated ovarian-hormone fluctuations may play a part in premenstrual syndrome, but none of the studies to date has proven this to be true.

In England and other parts of Europe, researchers have studied a new drug called bromocriptine, which inhibits the release of prolactin, but unfortunately these studies have shown little promise. The researchers initially thought that prolactin levels were higher in women with premenstrual tension, but they have learned that prolactin levels are probably normal in most of these women. Furthermore, women with pituitary tumors, which cause tremendous amounts of prolactin to be secreted, usually don't experience the symptoms of premenstrual syndrome.

In this country, Sandoz Pharmaceuticals markets bromocriptine as Parlodel. In most of the studies conducted by Sandoz in Europe, the therapeutic effects of Parlodel proved to be no different from those of placebo, although Parlodel is a potent drug with multiple side effects. It is currently marketed for some types of female infertility. Sandoz plans no American premenstrual-syndrome studies at this time.[10]

One more note before leaving prolactin. Phenothiazines

(a group of tranquilizers that includes compazine, phenergan, stelazine, and others) are known to increase prolactin levels. If indeed prolactin is even partially responsible for premenstrual distress, the use of these and other related tranquilizers might serve to worsen the syndrome.[11] And, as you know, tranquilizers are liberally used to sedate women during this time of the month.

Other researchers think that vitamin B_6 may play some role in premenstrual syndrome. B_6 came into vogue to combat the depression that often accompanied the use of oral contraceptives. Since they create a functional deficiency of B_6, many thought that a similar deficiency might exist in women with premenstrual syndrome, thus explaining their depression. Some studies have reported successful treatment with B_6,[12] but other studies have failed to confirm those findings.[13] So the question remains open.

It is difficult to postulate therapies for a syndrome for which the cause is unknown. It seems to me likely that the solution to premenstrual syndrome has not been found because we have been looking for a simple solution to a complex problem. There probably is no single hormone or chemical that is responsible for premenstrual syndrome, but I have long felt that prostaglandins are involved.

Most likely the symptoms are the result of a complex chain of events that goes something like this: cyclic variations in the hormones estrogen, progesterone, and prolactin occur, and the ratio of one hormone to another fluctuates. Changing hormone ratios lead to increased levels of secondary substances—very probably prostaglandins. Increased prostaglandin levels, in turn, affect the amount of chemical transmitters present in the brain and their activity. Neurotransmitter activity has a direct effect on mood; marked changes cause mood swings. And all the while, the prostaglandins themselves produce such physical symptoms as pain, tenderness, and nausea. At least, that is my theory.

The research so far has uncovered a great deal of information about prostaglandin levels during menstruation, but has not yet accurately measured or differentiated the various separate prostaglandin levels during the entire menstrual cycle, especially during the premenstrual week. No one knows if the ratios of one to the other are the same during these days as they are during menstruation.

We know that total prostaglandin levels increase during the latter part of the cycle and fall with menstruation, so they should be primary suspects for causing premenstrual-syndrome symptoms.

This theory also fits women who suffer from severe post-partum blues, since the tremendous levels of prostaglandin they have in their bodies during labor suddenly drop with delivery (as do the levels of estrogen and progesterone). The drop in prostaglandin plus an increase in prolactin may be all that is necessary in some women to completely botch up the brain chemistry for a few weeks.

The prostaglandin theory also makes sense to me because women with premenstrual syndrome have many symptoms that can be directly related to excess prostaglandin production. For example, they complain about joint pain or tenderness when they are premenstrual. We already know that patients who have arthritis have increased amounts of prostaglandins in their joint fluid.[14] Most premenstrual women have sensations of lower abdominal cramping for three to four days prior to the onset of their periods, and it has already been documented that prostaglandins cause uterine contraction. The headaches that many women suffer premenstrually have been shown in some cases to be brought on by prostaglandins. Bowel habit changes and general discomfort are also due to prostaglandins. We also know that breast tenderness is related to an increase in cystic fluid accumulation and higher prostaglandin production by these cysts.

Just to round things out—if you're still with me—prolactin increases prostaglandin production[15]—and so does another well-known culprit, caffeine. Ergot, a drug that is a potent blood vessel constrictor, has been shown to be effective in one study of premenstrual syndrome. Interestingly enough, it works by blocking prostaglandin manufacture.[16] There is recent evidence that prostaglandin levels are lowered when progesterone is given. This factor may account for some of Dalton's success.

In order to test my theory that prostaglandins contribute to premenstrual syndrome, and to see if the antiprostaglandins were as effective in relieving menstrual pain in women with maximal congestive symptoms, I set up an eight-month double-blind crossover study using the antiprostaglandin drug Ponstel, the same drug that had done so well in patients with spasmodic dysmenorrhea.

I adapted the questionnaires and study design from my previous dysmenorrhea study. (In retrospect, I feel that had I modified the questionnaires to better fit the problems of premenstrual syndrome, I would have gotten more reliable data. But then good study designs are often developed by trial and error.)

Forty-three women who had a variety of complaints about premenstrual days enrolled in the study. Most had breast tenderness, abdominal bloating, and premenstrual anxiety. Only a few had menstrual discomfort.

After the study had begun, I realized that there were only five women in the entire group who had monthly menstrual pain, too few for any valid scientific evaluation, though four out of the five did get relief. It was more interesting to pursue the notion that prostaglandins might cause the specific symptoms of premenstrual syndrome. For example, breast tenderness could be caused by excess amounts of prostaglandins that make the nerve endings more sensitive. Abdominal bloating, created by changes in gut motility and accumulations of fluid and gas, may be caused by prostaglandin shifts.

The mental premenstrual symptoms that some women experience are harder to explain. Changes in prostaglandin levels may be only one step in their development. Such changes could lead to other changes in the amount and activity of chemical messengers in the brain. These neurotransmitter substances (messengers) have a direct effect on our emotions, which may trigger symptoms such as irritability or lethargy. And so if premenstrual syndrome were caused in total or in part by prostaglandin increases, it followed that antiprostaglandin medications could relieve the symptoms.

I instructed all the women in the study to begin taking the study drug at the onset of their premenstrual symptoms and to take only the amount of medication that they needed, up to a maximum of four capsules per day for seven days. Half took Ponstel, half placebo for four months, then there was a crossover to the second substance. It is not always possible to judge when your period will come, so from time to time, women would only get in a day or two of medication because their menses would come early or because they calculated wrong. Therefore, the dosages of medication varied from month to month.

Utilizing statistical analysis tests to compare the Ponstel-treated patients with the placebo-treated patients, it was determined that: Ponstel patients showed a significantly greater relief of premenstrual breast tenderness, abdominal bloating, ankle swelling, menstrual pain, and less nausea associated with menstruation. There was no statistical improvement, however, in mental symptoms such as tension, lethargy, or depression.[17]

As far as I am aware, this was the first study in the world that was designed to evaluate the effect of an antiprostaglandin in the treatment of premenstrual syndrome. Although it could not be considered a complete success, small gains were made. To put it in perspective, it is important to understand that this study showed better results than nearly all the European studies done with progesterone or bromocriptine. Furthermore, antiprostaglandin medications have few side effects, especially compared to drugs such as bromocriptine.

Of further interest, since the end of the study, nearly half of the women have continued to take Ponstel for their premenstrual symptoms. Some women in the study continue to take the drug for abdominal bloating; others for nausea and cramping or other symptoms. Each women seems to have her own reason for continuing the medication.

One patient took it religiously for her breast tenderness. Forgetting it while on vacation, she returned and called to say that she had been miserable while she was away. Her breast tenderness was back to where it had been before the study, and she found it too painful to sleep on her stomach during her premenstrual days.

Another patient forgot her pills when she went to the Caribbean. Even though she was on vacation and away from her usual job pressures, she still felt very anxious and irritable during her premenstrual time.

Although there was no statistical improvement of anxiety or depression in the group as a whole, obviously some women felt that they had worthwhile results. Whether these women had different chemistries or simply imagined relief, I don't know.

So many areas in premenstrual syndrome remain to be investigated that many researchers should be encouraged to involve themselves with this task. Just the numbers of suffering women alone is reason enough to put this problem high on the agenda of the research community. There's a lot of work to be done, and millions of women are waiting.

As of now, there is no single treatment for premenstrual syndrome that has proven universally effective. Of the many therapies that have been introduced over the years with great enthusiasm—oral contraceptives, progesterone, diuretics, tranquilizers, vitamins, psychotherapy, lithium, bromocriptine—none has survived the all-important controlled, scientific, clinical trial.

Even though we have not yet found the single "magic bullet" that is effective for all women with premenstrual syndrome, there are some effective ways to treat its various symptoms. So let us put complicated theories aside for the moment and consider some specific symptoms and ways to alleviate them.

Of the many physical symptoms that can occur, the most common is bloating, usually apparent in enlarged, tender breasts and/or swelling of the abdomen. When bloating is severe, women complain of weight gain, but most women actually add only one or two pounds. (Rarely will a woman gain more than five pounds.)

Bloating is so common that water retention has been suspected as the prime cause of premenstrual syndrome, but studies find that there is no real difference in weight gain between those who suffer symptoms of premenstrual syndrome and those who don't, so water retention per se is not the primary cause.

In a study of twenty patients with severe premenstrual syndrome and twenty controls without symptoms, Andersch et al. found that in neither group were there significant changes in water or body weight in the premenstrual period.[18] Wong hypothesized that the symptoms of premenstrual syndrome may be due to a shifting of body fluid from the blood vessels and capillaries into the tissues. Such a shift from one place to another could occur without causing a difference in overall body weight.[19]

Abdominal distension could be due to such a fluid shift. It may be minimal and only noticed because tight pants no longer zip easily, or it may be much more pronounced and require larger-size pants for the week or so before menses. Women often note that they urinate less often during the premenstrual period, but at the onset of menses, urine production increases and a rapid dissolution of the bloatedness occurs.

Bloating and water retention can be relieved simply by reducing your salt intake for seven to nine days before your period. Reducing salt means more than just not adding salt to your food. It means cooking with less salt and avoiding foods that are high in sodium, such as commercial salad dressings, gravies, canned or dried soups, boullion, sauerkraut, olives, pickles, lox, ham, bacon, hot dogs, peanut butter, salted popcorn, and so on. Condiments and seasonings that contain salt, such as monosodium glutamate, Worcestershire sauce, and soy sauce, should not be consumed that week, either.

You can get around some of these constraints if you use flavorings such as pepper, garlic, onions, and herbs. Just remember to buy garlic powder, not garlic salt, and learn to make your own salad dressings and sauces. Any packaged soup will contain many milligrams of sodium, and so will most other foods prepared outside your own kitchen. So try to avoid packaged and canned foods at this time, or at least check the labels carefully for sodium content. Restaurant food, too, is universally highly salted, so try to avoid eating out that week.

The list of foods with high sodium content on page 89 will help you remove these items from your diet one week before you expect your period.[20] Also note low and moderate sodium foods on page 88.

Despite the relief to be obtained through these simple dietary changes, for years doctors have been treating women for premenstrual water retention with powerful diuretic drugs. They prescribe large doses of potent kidney-stimulating drugs originally meant to be used by patients with heart and kidney failure and severe hypertension. And so many women spend much of the day in the bathroom urinating quarts of salt and water. This process is supposed to make them feel better, but it often leaves them literally drained and exhausted. It may reduce some of the swelling, but it does little to alleviate irritability and often increases exhaustion.

Potent antihypertensive and diuretic drugs were designed for sick patients who commonly have swelling in the parts of their bodies that are most affected by gravity: their ankles, lower legs, and even their lower backs, should they be confined to bed. If their hands are down, their fingers swell. Such patients gain weight in five- and ten-pound increments.

Premenstrual women do not suffer these symptoms; their swelling is most prominent in the breasts and abdomen.

Foods with Low Sodium Content—may be used as desired unless calories are also restricted

ALL FRUIT AND FRUIT JUICES
ALL FRESH OR FROZEN VEGETABLES EXCEPT THOSE IN FOLLOWING LISTS

BREAD/
CEREALS:
Puffed wheat/rice or shredded wheat
Most hot, unsalted cereals
Salt-free breads
Pearl barley, rice, noodles, macaroni, spaghetti
Popcorn, unsalted

FATS:
Sweet butter   Salt-free mayonnaise
Unsalted margarine   Sour cream
Vegetable oils   Nuts, unsalted

MISC:
Vinegar   Honey and syrup
Wines   Sugar
Jams or jellies

Herbs and spices which do not contain salt or MSG (monosodium glutamate)

Special salt-free foods (read the label to determine milligram level per serving—under 15 mg per serving foods may be used as desired).

Foods with Moderate Sodium Content—must be limited in amounts as specified

MILK:
Limit to 2 cups daily

EGGS:
Limit to 1 per day

DESSERTS:
Limit to one choice per day—serving portion as indicated
Cake—1½ oz
Cookies, assorted—1 oz
Gelatin—½ cup
Ice cream—½ cup
Regular cooked puddings such as tapioca, rice, etc.—½ cup
Sherbet—½ cup

MEAT/FISH/
FOWL:*
(other than those in following list)—Limit to 6 oz cooked weight daily

VEGETABLES:
Limit to one choice per day—½ cup serving only (fresh, frozen or salt-free canned)
Beets   Frozen lima beans
Beet greens   Frozen peas
Carrots   Kale
Chard   Mustard greens
Dandelion greens Turnips, white
Celery

*Fresh crab, lobster, shrimp, scallops, brains, kidneys, and frozen fish which have been flumed in brine contain higher amounts of sodium than other fresh fish and meats. Those foods should be chosen infrequently.

Foods with High Sodium Content—should be avoided for seven to ten days before your period

MILK:	Buttermilk
CHEESE:	All excepting special low sodium cheese or low sodium cottage cheese.
MEAT/FISH/ FOWL:	Bacon, ham, frankfurters, sausages, bologna, luncheon meats; canned, salted, dried, smoked or pickled meat, fish or poultry. Herring, caviar, regular canned tuna and salmon, anchovies, sardines and salted cod. Canned crab, shrimp, lobster and oysters. Salt pork, chipped or corned beef, brain, kidney, meats koshered by salting. Regular peanut butter.
VEGETABLES:	Sauerkraut, olives, pickles, regular canned vegetables and canned vegetable juices. Any vegetable prepared in brine.
FATS:	Salted butter or margarine, commercial salad dressings and regular mayonnaise, bacon fat, salted nuts, canned gravies.
BREADS/ CEREALS:	Regular and yeast breads and rolls prepared with salt, dry cereals other than those in first list, regular pancakes, muffins, biscuits, cornbread, crackers and mixes. Potato chips, corn chips, pretzels, salted popcorn, etc. Quick cooking cereals if a sodium compound has been added in processing. Cornmeal and self-rising flour.
SOUPS:	All regular canned soups, soup mixes, broth, bouillon, consommé, commercial bouillon cubes, powders or liquids.
BEVERAGES:	Dutch process cocoa, soft drinks or beer which have been bottled in areas with high sodium content in their water supplies.
DESSERTS:	Instant puddings, pie crust unless prepared without salt, desserts in excess of the amount allowed in previous list.
CONDIMENTS:	Salt, seasonings which contain salt or monosodium glutamate, Worcestershire sauce, soy sauce, meat tenderizers, regular catsup, chili sauce, barbecue sauce, horseradish sauce, etc. Pickles, relishes and olives.

Carefully read the labels of all prepared foods. Look not only for salt, but also for bicarbonate of soda (baking soda), baking powder, MSG, and sodium compounds such as sodium benzoate and sodium citrate. Most frozen dinners, instant dinner mixes, sauces, canned foods (except fruits and fruit juices) and prepared foods contain salt unless they are especially prepared for sodium-restricted diets and labeled as such.

Water varies in sodium content from one area to another. Check with your local water supplier, and if the water in your area contains more than 20 mg sodium per quart, bottled water should be used. The use of water-softeners may add significant amounts of sodium to the water supply.

Avoid medicines, laxatives, and salt substitutes unless prescribed by physician.

They should not be treated as if they had heart or kidney failure. Since I feel strongly that such treatment is inappropriate, I have used only one diuretic in the past fifteen years to treat premenstrual syndrome—Dyrenium, or, generically, triamterene.

I chose Dyrenium because it works directly on the kidneys to get rid of salt (sodium) and water; unlike other diuretics, such as Hydrodiuril, Esidrix, or Lasix, it does not lower blood pressure and cause a loss of potassium. Premenstrual-syndrome patients don't need their blood pressure lowered since most of them are young and tend to have low blood pressure to begin with. Nor do I want them to suffer a potassium loss. The Andersch study found that for women suffering premenstrual syndrome, the single most important factor in the immediate premenstrual days was that they had too much water in proportion to their body potassium.[21] Treating such women with antihypertensive medications (diuretics), which lower potassium levels further, can only worsen the situation. In addition, low potassium levels produce feelings of weakness and lethargy, and those feelings are already prominent enough in premenstrual syndrome. Dyrenium, on the other hand, is the only diuretic I know of that was not meant to be an antihypertensive but only to get rid of fluids. And that's exactly what the premenstrual woman needs: sodium and water loss without potassium loss and without effect on her blood pressure.

Why don't more doctors use Dyrenium? When the drug salesman from its manufacturer (Smith, Kline and French) came into my office a few months ago, I asked him, "Why don't you ever try to sell me on Dyrenium?"

He looked at me a little sheepishly and said, "You know, it's not a very powerful drug, and though it gets rid of some fluid, it won't lower blood pressure. We don't push it very much and it doesn't sell too well."

I looked him straight in the eye and said, "But that's exactly what is so good about the drug—it's perfect for women with premenstrual syndrome for just those reasons that you think it's so awful. Premenstrual women don't need a powerful drug to lower their blood pressure; they just need a water pill to get rid of a little of their bloating. And Dyrenium won't upset their potassium balance. You guys have been missing the boat." As soon as the bewildered salesman left my office, I wrote Smith, Kline and French a letter and got the whole thing off my chest.

Because Dyrenium is mild, women often call me when they first begin taking it and say, "I used to spend the morning in the bathroom when I took Lasix; I haven't noticed anything today."

Then I will say, "But how do you feel?"

They usually say, "Okay."

That's all that's important. Furthermore, the excretion of sodium, which results in decreased fluid retention, cannot be measured by the amount of time one spends in the bathroom.

Aldactone (spironolactone), a diuretic and antihypertensive manufactured by Searle & Co., has been said to benefit women with premenstrual syndrome. It has been shown, however, to cause malignant tumors, including breast tumors, in rats. I therefore have chosen not to discuss this drug in this book, for I feel there are safer drugs available.

Women with premenstrual syndrome have been receiving drugs that are unnecessarily powerful and that cause greater salt imbalances in their bodies, which in turn begins a vicious cycle of need for constant diuretics. This dependence on daily diuretics is a serious problem. There is no reason to use an elephant gun to shoot a mouse. Premenstrual syndrome needs a mouse gun, one that is specifically tailored for the job and that won't cause more problems than it is supposed to solve.

Another common symptom of premenstrual syndrome is a terrible craving for sweets. This may be due to low blood-sugar levels (hypoglycemia), although, to date, the place of hypoglycemia in premenstrual syndrome—and even whether it is part of the syndrome at all—has not been documented. Writing in the *Irish Journal of Medical Science,*[22] Robert Bell notes that

> The symptoms of hypoglycemia are highly varied and are primarily psychological and neurological. The individual may feel faint, dizzy, weak, disturbed and nervous. The negative emotions include anxiety, depression, and impulsivity. Aggressiveness and irritability in one form or another are quite common. . . .
>
> The reasons for increased aggressive tendencies during hypoglycemia (low blood sugar) are not yet clear, although some of the effects of low blood glucose on the central nervous system give some indications. It is associated with epilepsy and with disruptions in EEG patterns.

Bell concludes that if, as in the case of alcohol, the brain systems first affected are the ones related to inhibition, then hyperaggressiveness might be expected to occur with hypoglycemia. Some feel that hypoglycemia may be the basis for irritability and aggressiveness associated with premenstrual tension.

The best remedy for premenstrual hypoglycemia is probably the usual regimen used to treat patients who have hypoglycemia all the time. It consists of frequent feedings— three meals plus three snacks per day—of low-carbohydrate, high-protein, and low-fat foods.

Fullness and tenderness in the breasts is another frequent premenstrual complaint: most of the swelling occurs along the upper outer portion of the breast, where most of the glandular tissue is located, and also in the area of the nipple. Some women have so much tenderness that the pressure of clothing becomes irritating. Sometimes sleeping with a bra on helps. For reasons yet unknown, some months bring more discomfort than others.

From time to time, a woman will appear in my office and state that her breasts are so tender that she cannot sleep. She is frightened and wants to know what is the matter.

After examining her and finding out that she is premenstrual, all I can say is that once in a while some women have a bad month. Their usual symptoms are greatly exaggerated for unknown reasons. This also happens to women with menstrual pain. They go along for three or four months with rather benign periods, requiring only an aspirin or two. Then for no apparent reason, not because of apparent increased stress or other psychological reasons, they have a terribly painful period. Our ability to understand this phenomenon is limited because we can't easily scientifically measure the various hormones, prostaglandins, or other substances that may be involved. Having observed these bad months in my patients over the years, I have developed suspicions of my own and a painless experiment—in which you can participate—to test my theory.

I believe that these bad months may be brought on simply by too much coffee, tea, cola, or chocolate. All these drinks contain caffeine or caffeinelike chemicals belonging to a class of compounds known as xanthines (or methylxanthines). Although the strength of the different xanthines varies, all have the same physiologic effects on the body.

Caffeine is a brain stimulant that can be used to overcome drowsiness and fatigue. In fact, it has the ability to nullify the effect of a tranquilizer or sleeping pill. This effect of caffeine and the other xanthines, however, is a double-edged sword because it also causes anxiety, insomnia, nervousness, irritability, and shakiness—symptoms virtually indistinguishable from those seen in premenstrual syndrome. In addition, xanthines can cause a rapid heart rate or irregular heartbeats. And coffee, whether decaffeinated or not, can cause nausea, vomiting, diarrhea, and occasionally ulcers. (This effect is caused by the irritating oils in the coffee and is not purely because of caffeine.)

Caffeine content varies among beverages and, in the case of coffee, varies greatly depending on the manner of preparation. The longer coffee or tea is brewed, or the finer the grind, the higher the caffeine content of the drink.

Colas differ greatly in the amount of caffeine they contain. The following table reflects the caffeine content of these beverages.[23]

	Beverage	Caffeine per 5-oz serving	100 ml
Coffee	instant, decaffeinated	3 mg	2 mg
	instant, regular	66	44
	percolated	110	73
	dripolated	146	97
Tea	bagged, black, 5-minute brew	46	33
	bagged, black, 1-minute brew	28	20
	loose, green, 5-minute brew	35	25
Chocolate Products	Cocoa	14	—
	Chocolate syrup, 2 table-spoons	14	—
	Small chocolate candy bar	20	—

	Caffeine per 12-oz can	
Coca-Cola	65 mg	18 mg
Dr Pepper	61	17
Mountain Dew	55	15
Diet Dr Pepper	54	15
Tab	49	14
Pepsi-Cola	43	12
Regular Sunkist Orange	40	11
RC Cola	34	9
Diet RC	33	9
Diet-Rite	32	9
Diet Sunkist	0.6	0.15
Root Beer	0	0

J. F. Greden in the *American Journal of Psychiatry* suggested that more than 250 milligrams of caffeine per day is excessive. That's less than the amount that you get from two cups of dripolated coffee. However, the effect of a given amount of caffeine depends upon body size and weight. If a child drinks a can of cola, Dr Pepper, or Mountain Dew, the caffeine intake is comparable to an adult drinking four cups of instant coffee. If a nursing mother drinks coffee, her milk will contain caffeine, which can have a stimulating effect on her baby.[24] Furthermore, the FDA has recently completed studies that implicate caffeine in causing birth defects. If these studies are further substantiated, warnings to pregnant women will appear on products containing caffeine.

I used to be a moderate user of xanthines. I drank two or three cups of coffee each day and a cup of tea with lunch. Then I read the studies of benign breast disease done by Dr. John Minton, who concluded that xanthines are responsible for the growth of breast cysts.[25] I decided to go off all caffeine, not because I had breast cysts but rather to see if there would be a change in my breast tenderness premenstrually. I reasoned that if xanthines contributed to the production of breast cysts, as Minton believes, then without xanthines, breast-cell activity in general would decrease and premenstrual syndrome might have one less bothersome symptom. Furthermore, if one symptom might be affected, others might also follow a common pathway.

And so I stopped drinking beverages that contain caffeine. I switched to Postum instead of coffee, but with lunch, I still have tea. I figured that since I like tea so very weak, there could hardly be enough caffeine in it to influence anything one way or another. I also convinced a few patients to experiment with me.

Generally, all of us felt that we had less breast tenderness. Those who had drunk more than four cups of coffee per day called me after switching to tell me that they had been less irritable and generally had a better month. I also think that my menstrual cramps have been much milder since I stopped ingesting caffeine. In fact, I require much less medication (one Ponstel in each of the last two months instead of three to four). One patient told me that her symptoms had improved, but she had gone back to coffee because she needed it to wake her in the morning. Just before she hung up, I asked her about her menstrual cramps and how much medication she had taken during the two months that she had been off coffee.

"Oh my God," she said, "I never realized until just now that I never needed any for the two months that I gave up coffee."

Another patient sent me a note that said,

> When you suggested that I go off coffee, tea, cola, and chocolate, it was quite a surprise. I only drank one to two cups of coffee per day, but you felt that I might be one of those women who was extremely sensitive to caffeine. You also put me on Dyrenium and a low-salt diet for a week before my period. That meant even though I did not have to stop teaching Chinese cooking, I couldn't eat any of the foods I prepared because they were always made with soy sauce or MSG. But whatever I gave up was worth it. I have had three months of saneness, after years of premenstrual horror. Not only do I love you, but my daughter, and most especially my husband send their thanks.

It is not possible to make any scientifically valid statements about the effectiveness of a no-caffeine treatment from this tiny sample. Nonetheless, this is an experiment that anyone can do for herself. After all, it's simple, costs nothing, and just might provide exactly the relief you need.

I am also undertaking a larger study of this phenomenon, since I am persuaded that caffeine and the other xanthines in some way make the symptoms of premenstrual syndrome more severe. For this reason, I wrote to Dr. Minton and suggested that he add questions about premenstrual syndrome to his patient questionnaire on breast cysts. He might then learn independently the effects of stopping the intake of xanthines on premenstrual syndrome.

If you achieve relief of your symptoms during the two months of abstinence, you may elect to continue to restrict your intake of xanthines. Total abstinence may not be necessary, and you may choose to experiment with decaffeinated coffee, a lesser amount of regular coffee consumption or some other beverage. My favorite is boiling water, juice of $\frac{1}{4}$ lemon and 2 teaspoons of sugar.

At the present time, such symptomatic relief is the best we have to offer, for we have not yet found the effective cure (or cures) for premenstrual syndrome as we have for menstrual cramps. Still, most women will be able to reduce their discomfort by treating their symptoms. To recapitulate, here are the procedures to follow:

1. Go on a low-sodium diet for seven to ten days before the onset of menses.
2. Drink no coffee, tea, cola, or chocolate. Some women find that one cup of regular coffee or two cups of de-caffeinated coffee per day does not affect them, so you may want to experiment to determine your own sensitivity. *Note:* this is every day, *not* just before menstruation.
3. If steps 1 and 2 do not do the trick, then take the diuretic Dyrenium (100 mg) daily after breakfast for seven or eight days prior to menses. Stop the diuretic the day you begin to flow. (You need a doctor's prescription for this.)
4. To combat fatigue and weakness, eat small, high-protein snacks every few hours and cut back on sweets and other high-carbohydrate foods.

Following these steps won't cure you, but it will make your premenstrual syndrome easier to live with. For now, that's the best we can do.

CHAPTER 3

Contraception:
Safe at Any Age

In this day and age, one would assume that the mature woman would know about all types of birth control from condoms to tubal ligation, but unfortunately, even sophisticated women all too often have frighteningly little knowledge about birth control. I remember appearing on a noontime television talk show in New York City with a hostess who was filling in while the permanent host was on vacation. As I talked about birth-control devices, I opened a compact containing a diaphragm. She fluttered her long false eyelashes, stared at the rounded dome in my palm, and said, "What in the world is that?" I paused, sat back, and discussed her question. Here was a sophisticated, intelligent woman with a successful career who had never even seen a diaphragm!

But I can also empathize with people in this situation. It frequently amazes me that I have done so many talk shows on contraception, because when I was age 15, I wasn't too sure that you could not get pregnant from kissing. When I was in medical school, I was rewarded with a frog in my purse for failing to recognize a condom as the "balloon" in one of our science-lab experiments. I never saw a diaphragm until I was asked to fit a patient with one. Luckily,

I was in practice at that time with another woman, who taught me what I needed to know, though not without some trial and error. I remember my first lesson and the three of us who took part—two female doctors and a young patient. I was trying to get the slippery, lubricated diaphragm ring into my amused patient when suddenly, like a taut rubber band, it slipped from my gloved fingers and went flying across the room. Almost every woman who has ever used a diaphragm has had a similar experience with the "flying saucer" phenomenon, but the doctor is supposed to know better. Luckily, my patient and my partner laughed as hard as I did.

So no matter how old the woman, no matter what her social or economic position, no matter whether she has six children or none, I assume that my patients know very little about birth control. I remember all too well how little I knew, so I don't expect very much from anyone else. At least, that's usually a safe beginning.

But it should be only a beginning, for if you are female, contraception is your business, like it or not. So far as I know, no group of men anywhere in the world has ever assumed a fair share of the responsibility for birth control and family planning. The reason is rooted in simple biological fact. Since it is women who become pregnant, we have been compelled to take very seriously the responsibility for bearing children—or not bearing them—while men may not be deeply concerned, particularly those men who are just passing through. Any man who is less than what used to be called a gentleman may deny paternity to get off the hook; but no woman, finding herself inadvertently pregnant, can pretend the baby isn't hers.

Our social attitudes, which so often are literally man-made, reinforce this female responsibility. We tend to hold the woman wholly responsible for an unwanted pregnancy, as though she had brought off the conception all by herself. And although we supposedly live in a sexually liberated age, we cling tenaciously to the old double standard: when an unmarried woman becomes pregnant, society still regards her condition as a well-deserved punishment. "Nice girls" are still not supposed to "fool around." In fact, society's attitude toward pregnancy is almost wholly dependent upon the marital status of the woman: what is a happy blessing for the married woman is a suitable punishment for the unwed mother.

Medical research, too—always so much more willing to tamper with the female body than the male—has concentrated on developing methods of contraception that apply to the woman; then, since the methods apply to her, it is she who must use them. Perhaps in a more egalitarian future society, responsibility for birth control will be shared more equally by women and men.

For now, learn all you can about contraception, if not for your own benefit, then certainly for your daughter's. Like it or not, America's adolescents are engaging in sex at a younger age. One-third of all women are sexually active by age 15, more than one-half by age 19. The illegitimate birth rate in the 15- to 19-year-old age group is increasing rapidly. By the time these young women present themselves at a clinic or doctor's office for contraception counseling, most of them have been engaging in sex for two to six years. Most have had from one to three partners, after starting in a monogamous relationship.

A study conducted at the Long Island Jewish Hospital[1] asked adolescent girls who came to the clinic for contraception why they had not used a contraceptive before. Their responses were:

Didn't know I'd get pregnant.	25%
Didn't worry about it.	23%
Afraid to ask.	23%
Too young to get it.	10%
Didn't know it was available.	8%

Seventy-two percent of these teenagers did not believe that they were risking pregnancy at the time of intercourse; half of them didn't know that there is a particular time of the month when they could become pregnant. Often, girls don't even know when they are pregnant. I examined one 16-year-old—a big, stocky, athletic girl—and found her to be in her ninth month. Her mother had brought her for an examination because she had a bad cold and frequent "gas pains." A week later she gave birth. For these uninformed, unfortunate girls, then, as well as for ourselves, we should learn all that we can about contraception.

The ideal contraceptive would offer 100 percent protection from pregnancy and be absolutely safe, constantly available, esthetically pleasing, and easily reversible, and would not require any planning. However, the ideal contraceptive does not exist, despite our impressive development of technology in so many other fields from communications to interplanetary travel; even though the search has been underway for centuries, the perfect contraceptive still remains to be found.

There are, however, many effective methods of contraception to choose from. And that is the good news for women about contraception: you have a choice. No single method is right for everyone, and it is equally doubtful that any single method is right for anyone throughout her entire sexually active life. But there definitely is a method that is right for any given woman at any particular time in her life. Not only do you have a number of effective methods to choose from, but you have many choices within any given method. Do not feel locked in to using any particular contraceptive. Your circumstances change as you go through life, and so should your methods of contraception.

Selecting the method that is right for you depends upon many factors: age, marital status, number of partners, whether you want more children, and last but not least, how attentive and motivated you are. This last factor is, perhaps, most important, because if you are a person who forgets or who says, "To hell with it tonight," *many* methods will be ineffective for you. The contraceptive you choose should be tailored to your life-style and personality and should change as your circumstances change.

COITUS INTERRUPTUS

Coitus interruptus is unprotected intercourse in which the contraception is provided by the male's withdrawal before he ejaculates. Of all methods of contraception, this is the least effective. It borders on being a nonmethod.

In order for coitus interruptus to work, the male must not only withdraw before ejaculation but must also insure that none of the ejaculate comes into contact with any part of the external female genitalia. This is much easier said than done. Many males cannot time their ejaculation well enough, while others forget to do so in the heat of passion or suddenly change their minds. And since sperm are present in secretions from the penis during intercourse, even if withdrawal is well timed, pregnancy may be caused by the "pre-ejaculate."

Coitus interruptus is thought to be the preferred method among teenagers (since it requires no embarrassing visits to doctors or drugstores, and no cash) and may account for the high pregnancy rate in that age group. In addition, since it provides no protection from sexually transmitted disease, the practice undoubtedly contributes to the epidemic of venereal disease among teenagers. Coitus interruptus is *not* a recommended method of contraception, and anyone who has practiced it successfully has more luck than brains.

THE RHYTHM METHOD

Within each menstrual cycle, there is a period of about five days during which a woman can conceive. This period begins shortly before ovulation (the release of an egg by the ovary), which occurs about fourteen days, give or take a day or two, *before* the menses. The egg will live for only two days unless it is fertilized by the male sperm, but sperm usually live for three days in the woman (although they have been known to survive for up to a week). Thus during that five-day period when there is an opportunity for a live egg and a live sperm to be at the same place at the same time, a couple engaging in unprotected intercourse has an ex-·cellent chance of producing an heir. Since few women have perfectly regular, unvarying cycles, it is impossible to predict exactly when ovulation will occur. But we can determine a longer period of time—usually about ten days—during which a couple may avoid pregnancy by abstaining from intercourse. Success with this method of keeping in rhythm with a woman's menstrual cycle depends upon accurately determining her fertile period and abstaining from intercourse during it.

There are ways to help determine that fertile period, but none of them is consistently accurate. One such procedure, called the calendar method, requires keeping a record of menstrual cycles for six to eight months and then calculating the unsafe period on the basis of that record. Ovulation occurs fourteen days, plus or minus two, before menses, and three additional days must elapse to insure that any sperm present in the woman have died. So, counting the first day of flow as day one, by subtracting nineteen from the number of days in the shortest cycle you have recorded, you can determine the first unsafe day of your average cycle. By subtracting ten from the number of days in your longest cycle, you can determine the last unsafe day. For example, if your shortest cycle was twenty-six days and your longest was thirty-one, days seven through twenty-one are unsafe for you, and you should not have unprotected intercourse during that time.

Another method of determining the end of the fertile period uses a thermometer, because the body temperature drops slightly immediately before and rises sharply immediately after a woman ovulates. This change in temperature, of between 0.5 and 1 degree Fahrenheit, if it is detected, gives a pretty accurate indication that ovulation has occurred. Since a nonfertilized egg will survive for only two days, unprotected intercourse should be safe three days after the temperature rises. That temperature variation is so small, however, that a special basal thermometer (which costs about $6) must be used; and the temperature must be taken, preferably rectally, at the same time every day—immediately upon awakening, before getting out of bed or smoking a cigarette.

Changes in temperature indicate that ovulation has occurred, but do not signal the beginning of ovulation, so to be perfectly safe, a couple should abstain from intercourse from the onset of menses to three days after ovulation. By combining the thermometer method with the calendar method (to determine the beginning of the fertile period), you can reduce the period of abstinence, but you will also increase the risk of pregnancy.

Another method of determining when ovulation occurs relies on the changes which the cervical mucus undergoes during each cycle. Immediately after menstruation, there is very little cervical mucus, but as the time for ovulation approaches, mucus increases and becomes cloudy and sticky. During ovulation, the mucus becomes clear and very slippery, very much like egg white; and after ovulation, it becomes cloudy and sticky once more while lessening in amount. Before menstruation, it again becomes clear and watery. The chemical composition of the mucus also changes during these periods in both acidity and glucose content. Thus it is possible to determine the time of ovulation by observing the mucus or by testing it with litmus paper for acidity or with a test tape for glucose content. The dry period after menstruation would be considered safe, as would the period before menstruation, when the mucus is clear and watery. Not all women, however, experience these changes during every cycle, and any vaginal infection will affect the mucus; so the cervical-mucus pattern is not a reliable indicator of the fertile period in nearly one-third of women.

The advantages of the rhythm method are:

1. It is the only method the Catholic Church permits its members.
2. It is inexpensive.
3. It uses no devices during intercourse which might interfere with sensation.

The disadvantages are:

1. It is one of the least reliable contraceptive methods and should never be used by a woman who must not become pregnant.
2. It requires long periods of abstinence.
3. It requires organization and motivation.
4. It cannot be used by a woman who has irregular cycles.
5. It provides no protection against sexually transmitted disease.

SPERMICIDES

Vaginal spermicides are made up of a sperm-destroying agent dispersed in an inert, bulky base that is heavy enough to block the opening of the cervix and prevent the entrance of any sperm not killed by the agent. They are available in many forms, from many manufacturers. There are foams, creams, jellies, suppositories, and even foaming tablets. They can be purchased in almost every drugstore without a prescription and range in price from $3 to $6.

Any spermicide can be used in conjunction with a condom. A diaphragm must be used with a cream or jelly. When used alone, spermicides are somewhat less effective, but they provide good protection, and for most women, using foam alone seems a lot easier than having a diaphragm fitted in a doctor's office. Used alone, a foam is usually preferable to a jelly or cream, because the foam spreads very rapidly and coats the cervix evenly, while the more viscous jellies and creams spread neither as rapidly nor as evenly.

In order to get proper protection from any spermicidal foam or cream, you must use it correctly. The spermicide must be placed deep in the vagina, near the cervix. Foams and creams come with plastic tamponlike applicators for this purpose. (Be sure to purchase the combination pack with the applicator initially. Refill packages, consisting of the spermicide alone, can be purchased subsequently at a lower cost.) All spermicides must be inserted not more than sixty minutes before intercourse, and should be reinserted for each subsequent intercourse. There should be an interval of two or three minutes between insertion and intercourse. After intercourse, you should not douche or wash out the spermicide for at least six hours.

Suppositories and foaming tablets work in exactly the same way, but between insertion and intercourse, a longer interval must be allowed—about ten minutes for foaming tablets, fifteen minutes for suppositories—because they need additional time to disperse. These tablets and suppositories are no more effective than foam, but they are easier to carry because they are small. (Some creams also come in individually wrapped disposable applicators, which are easy to carry in a purse.)

Spermicides protect not only from pregnancy but also from infection. Laboratory tests show that these products inhibit the growth of the organisms that cause gonorrhea and syphilis. In the only clinical study to date, regular users of Delfen cream had fewer cases of gonorrhea than nonusers. This protection, although it is far from foolproof, is important, for gonorrhea is thought to be a major cause of pelvic inflammatory disease, which can produce sterility. According to one estimate, as many as 100,000 young women in the United States become sterile each year as a result of gonorrhea infections. Spermicides also protect against less serious vaginal infections, such as the well known *Trichomonas* and *Monilia (Candida)*, and they break down the protective envelope that covers the common herpes virus, rendering it less able to infect.

Researchers are investigating other methods of using spermicides, such as a throwaway vaginal sponge and a medicated vaginal ring that will be impregnated with a spermicidal substance. When they are perfected, these products will give further choices in contraception.

A new study has implicated sperm-killing creams, jellies, and foams in birth defects and increased rates of spontaneous abortion. To begin with, however, you must remember that most women routinely and correctly using these products do not get pregnant. The data therefore apply only to those women who have method failure. Hershel Jick, M.D., et al in the April 3, 1981, *JAMA* reported an increased incidence of limb-reduction deformities, tumors, chromosomal abnormalities, and congenital misplacement of the urinary opening to the undersurface of the penis. The frequency among infants whose mothers had used spermicide was 2.2 percent; for those women not using spermicides it was 1.0 percent.[2] The study concluded: "If spermicides induce some of the congenital disorders described in this study, the effect might be produced by an action on sperm, ova, or the embryo itself. Obviously, spermicides can damage sperm directly; should a damaged sperm produce conception, abnormalities could result. Alternatively, spermicides might be absorbed into the bloodstream and produce direct damage to the ovum before conception. Another possible mechanism would be a direct deleterious effect on the embryo."[3] Rabbit and rat studies have shown that spermicides are absorbed from the vaginal wall into the blood and general circulation. Absorption studies in humans have not been done to date.

Although women who use barrier methods have prided themselves that these are the safest and most "natural methods," it is possible that they have been fooled. However, before alarming everyone, this study's data still have to be proved by follow-up studies which may or may not confirm these conclusions.

The advantages of spermicides are:

1. They are up to 94 percent effective when used correctly and faithfully.
2. They provide some degree of protection against sexually transmitted disease because of their bactericidal (bacteria-killing) and viricidal (virus-killing) activity.
3. They do not interfere with the pleasurable sensation of intercourse.
4. They provide lubrication.
5. They are easily portable.
6. They are available without consulting a physician.

The disadvantages of this method are:

1. It requires planning.
2. It can interrupt the spontaneity of sex.
3. Men object to the taste during oral sex.
4. Creams and jellies tend to drip and leak from the vagina. Foams are less messy, tend to leak less, and are generally more esthetically pleasing.
5. Spermicides may be associated with increased risks of congenital defects or spontaneous abortion if the method fails and the woman becomes pregnant.
6. Some men and women have an allergic reaction to certain spermicides, which can usually be remedied by switching brands.

CONDOMS

Condoms, the age-old standbys, are also called rubbers, sheaths, safes, prophylactics, and sometimes by the trade name of the manufacturer, for example, Trojans, Ramses, or Fourex.

The condom is a thin sheath made of latex or lamb membrane, which covers the penis and prevents sperm from entering the vagina. No one knows when it was first used, but it has been around for centuries. In 1564, its use was described by Fallopius, an Italian anatomist, who recommended a linen condom for the prevention of venereal disease. Long before Fallopius, the ancient Romans were fashioning condoms out of the intestines and bladders of animals for the prevention of venereal disease.

Until modern times, the condom was the only effective means of contraception. Consequently, down through the years, it has been the scapegoat for our prudish attitudes toward sex. Many states and cities passed laws prohibiting the sale of condoms, and many people still think of them as paraphernalia of prostitution. This attitude was reinforced when condoms were distributed to soldiers as part of their prophylactic kits, not to protect women from pregnancy but to protect soldiers from VD. Since the condom has such a shady reputation, many people feel uneasy about using it.

Nevertheless, the condom remains one of the most reliable and safest contraceptives available. Many studies have shown that when it is properly and consistently used, it is 97 percent effective in preventing pregnancy. In addition, the condom protects best against sexually transmitted disease and may even offer protection from cervical cancer. Some researchers suspect that sperm may be a factor in causing cancer of the cervix, particularly among young women whose cervical structure is not yet stable and is most vulnerable to the potent chemicals (histones) that the sperm contain. The condom effectively prevents sperm from coming in contact with the cervix (see page 248).

Condoms are sold in drugstores and often in vending machines in men's lavatories. They come lubricated or non-lubricated, with or without a small reservoir on the end to hold the ejaculate, perfectly smooth or ribbed or knobby, colored or plain. They cost between $1 and $2, depending on the features chosen, for a package of three. They are usually individually wrapped and are easily carried in a wallet or purse. They can be used only once. Depending on the type chosen, the annual cost of contraception with condoms will be between $25 to $150, which makes them one of the more expensive methods of birth control.

To use a condom, place the rolled condom at the tip of the erect penis and unroll it down the entire length of the penis. An unlubricated condom may break because of friction during intercourse when normal vaginal lubrication is not sufficient, but prelubricated condoms may contain too much lubricant. If you are lubricating your own, as many people prefer, you should not use Vaseline or cold cream, which weakens the latex rubber. K-Y jelly, Surgilube, or a new product, Personal Lubricant, may be used, as they are water soluble, wash away easily, and will not affect the latex.

The penis should be withdrawn promptly after ejaculation

while the ring of the condom is firmly grasped to prevent spillage. Check the condom after use to be sure it has not ruptured. If it has broken, you should immediately fill your vagina with a contraceptive foam or douche with lukewarm water; and since neither of these methods is reliable, you may also want to consult your physician. The condom should be discarded in a wastepaper basket; never flush it down the toilet because it can clog the plumbing.

When it is properly used, the condom has a small rate of failure resulting from manufacturing defects such as pinholes or weakness in the sheath, from which ejaculate can leak. Consequently it is sometimes recommended that foam be used in conjunction with the condom, especially at midcycle. This combination method is nearly 100 percent effective and is equal in effectiveness to the pill; I often recommend it to women who can't take the pill but must have total protection from pregnancy.

The major dissatisfactions with the condom are:

1. It interrupts the spontaneity of sex, since it must be put on immediately before relations.
2. Men, and some women, find that it reduces their sensitivity and pleasure.
3. Users are aware of its presence, and some women, as well as men, dislike this fact.
4. Prompt withdrawal is necessary to avoid spillage.
5. Fear that the condom may slip off or break can result in less energetic lovemaking.

Interestingly enough, many couples find that these characteristics are sources of satisfaction for them. They report that the placing of the condom over the penis, when done by the female, is very sexy; the decrease in sensitivity results in prolonged intercourse; and awareness of its presence provides peace of mind.

The condom's advantages:

1. It is easy to use.
2. It is convenient.

3. It prevents infection.
4. It produces no side effects, except in the case of rare allergies to latex rubber or lubricants.
5. It does not require the intervention of a physician either to prescribe or fit.

THE DIAPHRAGM

The diaphragm is a circular, dome-shaped device made of latex rubber stretched over a thin metal ring. (The latex rubber is of much heavier gauge than that in the condom.) There are several manufacturers of diaphragms, but only four basic styles, which differ mainly in the type of metal ring that is used. The diaphragm is reusable and, with proper care, will last for up to eighteen months. It must always be used with a spermicidal jelly or cream, however, because it is ineffective alone. The diaphragm covers the cervix, and its main function is to hold the spermicide in place against the cervical opening.

The woman who wants to use a diaphragm must be fitted for the proper size by a physician or paraprofessional. She must also be trained to prepare, insert, and care for it.

A tube of spermicidal jelly or cream costs less than $5 and usually will provide enough spermicide for about ten applications. The diaphragm itself can be purchased at any drugstore for less than $10. Thus the annual cost of using a diaphragm is between $50 and $60 (not including your visits to the doctor). Diaphragms are sold in plastic cases that make them easy to carry in a purse or leave in a drawer.

It takes me two visits with a patient before she learns to use her diaphragm properly. During the first visit, I fit the diaphragm by trying a number of different-size fitting rings (the rims of the diaphragms only), and then I teach my patient how to use it. I try to find the largest possible size that is comfortable for her, because the vagina tends to expand with sexual excitement; using the largest possible correctly fitting size insures that the diaphragm will not be displaced during intercourse.

The spermicide is placed in the center of both sides of the dome of the diaphragm and spread around the edges. The diaphragm is then inserted, either by using an inserter or the fingers alone. It must be placed in the proper position behind the symphysis pubis, a bony shelf that serves to hold it in place. If the diaphragm is too small and does not fit snugly, it will slip far back into the vagina. If it is too large, it will hurt. And in either case—too small or too large— it will not provide good contraception. Unfortunately, diaphragms are sometimes poorly fitted—in most cases fitted too small. I am sure that this, along with "forgetting to use it," accounts for the majority of "diaphragm babies."

Once she has been fitted and given instructions, my patient goes home and practices putting in the diaphragm. When she is confident that she is doing it correctly, she returns to the office either wearing it or ready to put it in by herself in the office. We check it together to make sure she knows how to place it and how to make sure it is correctly positioned. When the diaphragm is inserted properly, fitting snugly behind the pubic bone, it is not possible to feel the back rim of the diaphragm. By inserting the entire second finger or second and third finger into your vagina, you can feel your cervix deep in the vagina—it feels like the tip of your nose—and make certain that the rubber dome of the diaphragm is covering the cervix and holding the sperm-killing cream or jelly in place. If your cervix is not covered by the diaphragm, you have no protection. When my patient has learned to place her diaphragm correctly and to double-check its position—then, and only then—she has my okay to use it.

The diaphragm is not effective if inserted more than two hours before sexual relations, because the spermicides lose their effectiveness. However, if coitus is delayed for more than two hours, simply inserting more spermicide into the vagina—without removing the diaphragm—will provide contraceptive protection. Additional spermicide must be added for each successive intercourse, and the diaphragm must remain in place for at least six hours after the last intercourse, which most often is overnight. When intercourse occurs in the morning, the diaphragm must be left in all day, and constant leaking from the vagina may make it necessary to wear a sanitary pad throughout the day.

The advantages of the diaphragm are:

1. It is 90 to 94 percent effective when properly used.
2. It does not interfere with the sensation or pleasure of intercourse (though some couples would disagree with this).
3. Some men and women may be allergic to the rubber or the spermicide and may complain of a burning sensation. Usually changing to a plastic diaphragm or a different brand of spermicide corrects the problem.
4. It may provide a degree of protection against sexually transmitted disease because of the bactericidal activity of the spermicide used in conjunction with the diaphragm.

The disadvantages of the diaphragm are:

1. It requires planning.
2. It is not readily available. (Although it is easily transported in your purse, if you leave it at home, it may be difficult to find a replacement in a hurry.)
3. It can interfere with the spontaneity of sex.
4. Not all women can use a diaphragm because of anatomic peculiarities.
5. If it is not properly fitted, it may contribute to recurrent bladder infections.
6. The spermicide used in conjunction with a diaphragm may be associated with increased risks of congenital defects or spontaneous abortion if the method fails and the woman becomes pregnant.

INTRAUTERINE DEVICES (IUDs)

One of the IUDs introduced in the United States several years ago was the Dalkon Shield. The design of this device made it very painful to insert and to remove. What's more, after it had been in use for a short time, doctors noted that a number of women who became pregnant while the Dalkon Shield was in place developed life-threatening infections. Eventually it was determined that the multifilamentous tail (made up of multiple filaments), which was encased in a sheath, was the cause of the infection, and not the IUD itself. The tail of the Dalkon Shield created a way for bacteria to enter and ascend into the sterile uterine cavity and cause infection. If the IUD failed to work and the woman became pregnant, her uterus, as it grew in size, drew the contaminated string up into its cavity. This tragedy, although it was rare, gave all IUDs a bad name and frightened many women away from using them. Even though the Dalkon Shield is no longer on the market, and all currently available IUDs have a safe, monofilamentous tail, the problem made all IUDs seem unacceptable and their use declined from a high of 10 percent to a current 7 percent of all women using contraception in the United States.

In many respects, this is a pity, because the IUD is a safe means of contraception that offers more benefits than risks to many women.

IUDs are as safe as birth-control pills for nonsmoking young women, and many times safer than the pill for older women. Using an IUD is five to ten times safer than childbirth.

The intrauterine device (IUD) is placed in the uterine cavity and provides uninterrupted contraceptive protection until it is removed. IUDs prevent pregnancy by preventing the implantation of the fertilized egg in the uterine cavity. IUDs come in many shapes, such as loops, coils, sevens, and Ts. Modern IUDs are made of flexible plastic of about the thickness of a piece of spaghetti and are generally about 1½ inches long.

Years ago, it was necessary to dilate the cervix—an extremely painful process—in order to insert a coiled or bent IUD. Modern IUDs were made possible by the development of new polymer plastic, a biologically inert material that has the property of "memory": once it is molded to a specific shape, it may be twisted thereafter and yet always returns to its original shape. This property makes it possible to straighten out the IUD for easy insertion, after which it returns to the initial conformation.

In order to be effective, inert plastic IUDs must have a size and shape that creates foreign-body reaction in the lining of the uterus, causing it to become slightly irritated. This irritation produces more white blood cells in the environment than usual, and scientists theorize that it is this condition that discourages the implantation of an egg, should it become fertilized. Some IUDs also contain material that has contraceptive properties. These medicated IUDs are smaller, because they do not depend on size for their effect. In fact, these IUDs, without their medication, depending upon size and shape alone, would be only 80 to 85 percent effective as contraceptives. With their medication, however, they are between 97 and 98 percent effective. They are generally more effective than inert IUDs, particularly the smaller sizes of inert IUDs.

The additional mechanisms that medicated IUDs rely on for preventing pregnancy are copper or progesterone. Copper is used in some because it interferes with cellular-enzyme systems that help the egg implant. It also causes an increase in the number of white blood cells present in the uterine cavity. Copper may also interfere with sperm mobility.[4] Progesterone causes the uterine lining to be slightly out of phase and not suitable for implantation of a fertilized egg. It may also make the cervical mucus more sticky, so that sperm cannot easily pass into the uterus. The small amount of progesterone released by the IUD does not affect ovarian function and cannot be detected in the bloodstream.

Some of the following data are from the manufacturers' inserts for physicians, and some came from studies. None of the numbers are gospel, for different studies done by different centers on the same type of IUD have yielded different results.

IUD Type	Pregnancy Rate per 100 Women used for 12 mo.	24 mo.	36 mo.	Expulsion 12 mo.	Medical Removal 12 mo.
LIPPES LOOP					
Size A	5.3	9.7		20.6	not given
Size B	3.4	6.3		19.6	
Size C	3.0	4.8		16.2	
Size D	2.7	4.2		12.7	15.2
COPPER-7	1.8	2.75	3.35	6.4	11.7
PROGESTASERT	1.8			3.1	12.2
TATUM-T	2.6	4.7	5.9	7.9	12.2
SAF-T-COIL*					
Size 25 S	—	—		—	—
Size 32 S	—	—		—	—
Size 33 S	2.8	3.1		18.3	15.6

*Good data on small sizes of Saf-T-Coil are not obtainable. They must be assumed to be poorer than the above data given for the largest size (33 S), used in women who have borne children.

Since there are so many different IUDs on the market, you should learn all you can about them and participate in the selection of the IUD that you receive. Beware of physicians or clinics offering only one type of IUD to all their patients, for no device is suitable for every woman. Each has advantages and disadvantages.

Inert IUDs are generally larger than medicated IUDs and tend to produce more pain and bleeding than you normally have during your menstrual periods. The copper-medicated IUDs (the Copper-7 and the Tatum-T) also increase bleeding, but to a lesser extent than the Lippes Loop. On the other hand, the Progestasert decreases heavy menstrual flow and lessens the pain of dysmenorrhea, though it may cause more intermenstrual spotting. Medicated IUDs have the disadvantage of needing more frequent replacement because the contraceptive substances added to them dissipate over time. The Copper-7 or Tatum-T must be replaced every three years. The Progestasert is replaced every year. (Alza, the manufacturer of Progestasert, has recently received preliminary approval from the FDA for women to use their current Progestasert for eighteen months.) Inert IUDs may be left in place for five years. Left in place for a longer time, an IUD may become weak and tend to break or may collect a gritty coat of calcium, which can irritate the uterine lining and may cause increasingly heavy bleeding. (This problem is easily remedied by removing the IUD and, if it is desired, inserting a new one.)

For women over thirty-five, who should not use the pill, the Progestasert IUD is especially well suited. The progesterone it contains helps maintain the correct hormonal balance in the uterine lining. Its required annual replacement, although not an incentive to its use, assures that the patient's Pap and pelvic exams, so important for mature women, will also be done annually. For these women, any IUD is a better choice than the pill, and I'm persuaded that it is also a better choice than tubal ligation because of the potential surgical complications involved in that procedure.

Some women should not consider IUDs at all. Any woman with any of the following conditions cannot have an IUD:

pregnancy
abnormalities of the uterus resulting in distortion of the uterine cavity
unusual or unexplained uterine bleeding
suspected cancer of the reproductive tract
acute Pelvic Inflammatory Disease (PID) or history of PID
Infected abortion or infection of the uterus following childbirth in the past three months
acute infection of the cervix (insertion must be delayed until infection is controlled)
previous ectopic pregnancy (occurs in a fallopian tube)
significant anemia (would not be a contraindication for a Progestasert)
chronic steroid therapy (because organisms might be introduced at the time of insertion)
Wilson's disease or allergy to copper (only pertains to copper-bearing devices)
valvular heart disease
leukemia

If you select an IUD and have none of these contraindications, the device can be inserted at any time, but the
ideal time is during or immediately after menstrual flow.
At that time, the physician can be sure that you are not
pregnant, and the opening to the uterus will be enlarged,
making the insertion easier and less painful. Furthermore,
the slight spotting that normally occurs with the insertion
of an IUD will not be noticeable or annoying while you
are menstruating.

The actual insertion of the IUD takes just two to three
minutes. There are several steps which should be meticulously followed. One of the important steps is "sounding"
the uterus. This is done by inserting a slender solid rod
into the uterus to measure the depth of the uterine cavity
and determine the direction and location of the uterine opening. Some physicians take short cuts and omit doing this.
This step, however, is critical because if the cervical opening
is too small or the uterine cavity is tiny and measures less
than 6.5 cm in depth the risk of pain, expulsion, or perforation is high. No IUD should be inserted if the measurements are less than 6 cm. Sounding also acquaints the
physician with any oddities of your uterine cavity and fore-
warns him of dangers or difficulties prior to actual insertion.
Insertion of an IUD without such knowledge, to my thinking,
is malpractice. Ask the person inserting your IUD if he will
be "sounding" your uterus—ask for the measurements if
you like.

Most women feel a few cramps during insertion. These
usually subside in a few minutes and completely disappear
in about half an hour. Some women experience discomfort
for a few hours. A woman having an IUD inserted should
expect her current period to be slightly heavier, more cramping than normal, and longer lasting. For the next two or
three cycles, she may note between-period spotting; or her
next period may come early (the full flow probably will come
on time, but she may spot two or three days early). IUDs
act locally within the uterine cavity, in contrast to birth-
control pills, which shut off the entire hormonal reproductive

system and affect almost every cell in the body. The patient with a newly inserted IUD should return to the doctor's office after her next menstrual flow to make sure the device has not been dislodged and no other problems have arisen.

Certain special situations may also call for the insertion of an IUD. For instance, insertion of a copper-containing IUD immediately after an unprotected intercourse can prevent implantation of the egg and forestall pregnancy. The IUD is effective for this purpose only if it is inserted within two to three days after ovulation; and the sooner after unprotected intercourse the insertion occurs, the better. If it is done in time, this procedure provides a better solution to unwanted pregnancy than abortion or the "morning-after" pill containing DES (diethylstilbesterol), with its unacceptable hormonal risks. An IUD might also be called for when a patient cannot be responsible for her actions because of mental retardation, or simply when she cannot be relied upon to take her pills, insert foam or a diaphragm, or insist that her partner use a condom. In this situation, the problem of pregnancy is more serious than the risk of venereal disease. However, it must be remembered that venereal disease may cause bigger problems when an IUD is in place.

Sometimes IUDs have to be removed for medical reasons, such as pelvic pain or cramping, excessive or abnormal bleeding, acute pelvic inflammatory disease that doesn't respond to antibiotics, displacement of the IUD from the uterus, pregnancy, or uterine or cervical malignancy. Women who want to become pregnant simply have their IUDs removed; and women who become menopausal should have the device removed within six months, since removal becomes more difficult as menopause progresses. Medicated IUDs must be removed and replaced at the appropriate time. In any case, removal takes only a few seconds and produces little discomfort. The doctor just pulls on the tail of the device and it slides out. This can be done at any time of the month, but if a new device is to be inserted during the same office visit, it should be scheduled to coincide with menstruation.

After removal, fertility is usually restored quickly. One

of my patients who wanted to have a baby asked me to remove her Copper-7. She called back in two weeks and said that she was pregnant. I was somewhat skeptical, but her pregnancy test in my office proved positive. She must have conceived with the IUD in place, and by the time the fertilized egg had moved down the fallopian tube and into the uterus, the device had been removed and normal implantation took place. The ability of her uterus to receive an egg was obviously restored immediately with the removal of the device, but I usually ask my patients to wait a month before trying to conceive, for then the uterine lining may be more "normal."

IUDs are ideal for women who always forget and for women who don't want to hassle at "that time." No other means of birth control demands so little from a woman. Once the IUD is inserted, the only thing to remember is to check once a month, after your menses, that the string, or tail, of the device is still present. This is done by simply inserting a finger high into the vagina and feeling the tiny thread that extends about an inch out from the opening of the cervix. Feeling the string is not always as easy as it may sound, because it is fine, and when warmed and moistened by the body, it is fairly imperceptible. Other than this once-a-month procedure (which takes about one minute), there is nothing else to do.

Women using an IUD who are unaccepting of anything less than 100 percent effectiveness (and 97 to 98 percent effectiveness is not to be sneezed at) can use a spermicidal foam during the middle of the month to cover the five or so fertile days.

Most women are delighted with the IUD and wish that they had always had such a convenient method of contraception. However, there are women who have had problems with their IUDs and hate them.

The most frequent inconvenience that IUD users encounter is increased bleeding—heavier flow or prolonged periods or spotting in between—sometimes accompanied by cramps or lower back pain.

With unmedicated devices such as the Lippes Loop C or D or Saf-T-Coil, menstrual blood loss measured at various intervals after insertion is approximately doubled over normal or preinsertion levels. With Copper-7 or Tatum-T devices, menstrual bleeding is also increased, but by a smaller amount.[5] This increased menstrual blood loss may put the user of copper and unmedicated IUDs in danger of anemia. In addition, it is inconvenient, annoying, and can be associated with increased menstrual pain. Progestasert, on the other hand, reduces the volume of menstrual bleeding up to 50 percent below preinsertion levels. It also decreases menstrual cramps. But like other IUDs, it may prolong the number of days of flow. Progestasert tends to cause more intermenstrual spotting, especially in young women.

Menstrual pain caused by an IUD, however, can be alleviated with drugs that inhibit prostaglandin synthesis—the same drugs that I use to treat primary dysmenorrhea. As I reported in the August 1979 issue of the *Journal of the American Medical Association*,[6] mefenamic acid (Ponstel), which I used in my dysmenorrhea studies, successfully alleviated pain caused by IUDs and also gave relief from such related symptoms as leg ache and backache. The increased menstrual flow that occurs because of IUDs also can be decreased by taking Ponstel or Motrin during the one to three days of maximal flow.

A more ominous complication of the IUD is infection of the female organs, called pelvic inflammatory disease (PID), which can lead to sterility. A broad-spectrum antibiotic is usually effective against PID. If this treatment does not provide relief in twenty-four to forty-eight hours, the IUD should be removed.

Whether PID is a complication of IUDs or just a fact of life is being debated in IUD circles. Jack Lippes recently argued that:

When IUDs first came on the American scene, in the 1960s, they were only used in women who had already had children and were married. In the 1970s, we saw a 400 percent increase in gonorrhea in this country. This was also the period when copper IUDs came on the market, and also Progestasert. Because of the smaller sizes of these devices, women received them who were single. The younger population is where the incidence of pelvic infection is greatest. The IUDs have not caused an increase in PID, but simply have been implicated by association.[7]

Studies have shown that the incidence of PID is significantly higher during the first two months following the first insertion of an IUD than during subsequent months. A large proportion of these early cases occurred in women who had a history of PID. Thus women who have had PID in the past are prone to having an acute PID flareup triggered by the IUD. Such women should consider other methods of contraception as their first choice and should inform their physician of their past PID experience.

The instructions that come with the Tatum-T acknowledge the danger. They state:[8]

An increased risk of PID associated with the use of IUDs has been reported. While unconfirmed, this risk appears to be greatest for young women who are nulliparous (childless) and/or who have a multiplicity of sexual partners. Salpingitis can result in tubal damage and occlusion, thereby threatening future fertility. Therefore, it is recommended that patients be taught to look for symptoms of PID. The decision to use an IUD in a particular case must be made by the physician and patient with the consideration of a possible deleterious effect on future fertility.

Symptoms of pelvic infection to watch out for are listed as: new development of menstrual disorders (prolonged or heavy bleeding), abnormal vaginal discharge, abdominal or pelvic pain, dyspareunia (painful intercourse), and fever. The symptoms are especially significant if they occur following the first two or three cycles after insertion.

The IUD also can break through the wall of the uterus into the peritoneal (abdominal) cavity, but such perforation occurs in less than one-tenth of 1 percent of users, and almost always at the time of insertion, when it may be accompanied by sudden pain or bleeding. If perforation occurs, an IUD containing copper should be removed immediately, because it can cause the formation of intra-abdominal inflammation and adhesions. Nonmedicated and progesterone-containing IUDs, although they should be removed as soon as is convenient, cause comparatively little reaction. Often their removal is accomplished through a laparoscope.

Pregnancy occurs in one to six IUD users per hundred per year, making IUDs second only to sterilization and the pill in contraceptive effectiveness. But the woman who becomes pregnant with an IUD in place faces added complications. When pregnancy results from IUD failure, removal of the device may end the pregnancy by precipitating spontaneous miscarriage. On the other hand, should the woman desire to continue the pregnancy and the device cannot be removed without causing miscarriage, there is increased danger of infection to her as well as to the fetus, because the IUD remains. While many women have completed pregnancy with an IUD in place, the risks of spontaneous miscarriage and septic (infected) mid-trimester miscarriage are increased.

Some studies indicate that IUD users, especially Progestasert users, run a higher than normal risk of tubal pregnancy, but these results have been challenged on the ground that the comparison group differed from the IUD users in ways that affect the risk of ectopic pregnancy. For example, the risk of ectopic pregnancy increases with age and is higher for women with a history of previous ectopic pregnancy or pelvic infection. One investigator (Sivin) concluded that

> The IUD could not have been a major factor contributing to the recent doubling in the rate of ectopic pregnancy in the United States.... With less than 10 percent of United States women of reproductive age using IUDs, clearly other factors are chiefly responsible for the rising incidence of ectopic pregnancy.[9]

The issue, however, has not been settled. Progestasert will have its package insert changed to make physicians and patients aware of this problem. It is important to remember that IUDs were designed to prevent intrauterine, not tubal, pregnancies.

Inert plastic IUDs are only the beginning of the evolution of the IUD. They have probably been produced in most of the possible configurations. As newer devices evolve, they will undoubtedly contain medications that reduce bleeding and cramping (possibly a small amount of an antiprostaglandin), as well as medications that will reduce herpes and other viral or bacterial infections (possibly copper and zinc). IUDs will become delivery systems that provide intrauterine therapies to those women who would benefit from locally placed medication. Currently being tested also are biodegradable IUDs intended to dissolve at a slow, predictable rate and obviate the need for later removal. In the future, then, even more choice will be available.

At the present, we can say that the advantages of an IUD are:

1. Once inserted, it requires little attention or concern.
2. It is one of the most effective contraceptive methods.
3. Since it acts locally in the uterus, it produces fewer side effects than the pill and is safer.
4. It does not interfere with spontaneity or sensation during intercourse.

The major disadvantages are:

1. It can cause heavy bleeding and cramping and anemia (except for the Progestasert IUD).
2. It can contribute to pelvic inflammatory disease.
3. It can become displaced in such a way—perforation or embedding—as to cause serious trouble to the user.
4. It requires the supervision of a physician.
5. It may contribute to the occurrence of ectopic pregnancy.

Mortality associated with pregnancy and childbirth, legal abortion, oral contraceptives (by smoking status) and IUDs, by age[10]

Age (years)	Pregnancy and Childbirth*	Legal Abortion†	ORAL CONTRACEPTIVES‡		IUDs‡
			Nonsmokers	Smokers	
15–19	10.4	1.0	0.6	2.1	0.8
20–24	9.5	1.4	1.1	4.2	0.8
25–29	12.1	1.8	1.6	6.1	1.0
30–34	22.8	1.8	3.0	11.8	1.0
35–39	43.7	2.7	9.1	31.3	1.4
40–44	68.2	2.7	17.7	60.9	1.4

*Per 100,000 live births (excluding abortion)
†Per 100,000 first-trimester abortions
‡Per 100,000 users per year

THE PILL

Oral contraceptives (the pill), which were approved by the Federal Drug Administration (FDA) for use in this country in 1960, are the most popular method of contraception in the world. In 1977, 325 million cycles—enough to supply 25 million women for one year—were sold.[11] Recently sales have been falling off in the United States and western Europe but are increasing in South America and Asia.

I expect that high-dose birth-control pills as we use them today will be withdrawn from use in the next five years. Current oral contraceptive therapy bathes all the body's cells with large amounts of powerful hormones in order to inhibit ovulation. These hormones effectively shut off the hypothalamus and pituitary glands; and when these glands do not secrete their hormones, the ovary does not receive a message to produce an egg and ovulation does not occur. The hormones in the pill also have a direct effect on the uterine lining, or endometrium, which causes it to become thin and to reduce its secretions. They also lower the receptivity of the cervical mucus to sperm and alter the function of the fallopian tubes.

The synthetic estrogen in birth-control pills is not comparable to the natural hormone because of its side effects and because it is given at a constant level for twenty-one days, in contrast to the fluctuating levels that occur with normal ovarian function. Newer birth-control pills contain lower doses of estrogen than earlier pills did, but since they still operate by suppressing ovulation, the dose of estrogen remains high enough to disrupt the normal hypothalamic-pituitary-ovarian relationship. In fact, birth-control pills shut down the entire female reproductive system.

Nevertheless, most women consider the birth-control pill a convenient method of contraception, especially when pregnancy is totally unacceptable. Oral contraception provides nearly 100 percent control and has been the method of choice for fifty million women worldwide. Free from the pressures of unwanted pregnancy, a woman has been able to enter college or the business world with a virtual guarantee that her career or education will not be interrupted.

The benefits from oral contraception are clear, but do they outweigh the risks? Bothersome side effects have been apparent since the introduction of the pill. These include nausea, vomiting, breast tenderness, and weight gain. In the past, weight gain was attributed to overeating, because it was felt that women on the pill were enjoying themselves more and worrying less. However, we have learned that the synthetic progesterone in birth-control pills has a direct effect on the appetite center of the brain and causes some women to gain weight.[12] The synthetic estrogen and progesterone in the pill are metabolized in the liver, and this increased activity may contribute to liver complications resulting in jaundice, tumors (both benign and malignant), abnormal production of liver proteins, and changes in cholesterol and triglycerides. Changes in carbohydrate metabolism are manifested in some women by the annoying occurrence of the common vaginal infection *Monilia vaginitis.* Rises in blood pressure have been noted to be from two and a half to five times the normal rate in women taking the pill; and pill takers develop gallstones at twice the normal rate after four years.

The blood of women taking the pill tends to clot easily,

putting them at a greater risk of heart attack and blood clots (which could occur anywhere in the body), especially in the over-30 age group. A study of forty-six thousand English women completed by the Royal College of General Practitioners found that women who used oral contraceptives for five years or more faced a tenfold risk of death from circulatory disease over women who have never used the pill.[13] Women on oral contraceptives who undergo major surgery have been found to have six times the number of thromboses. (Because of these findings, women scheduled for elective surgery should be taken off oral contraceptives for one month prior to surgery; and emergency surgery should be preceded by treatment with drugs to prevent clots.)

Because of the many side effects of oral contraceptives, women must return to their physicians for close follow-up. When I begin a patient on birth-control pills, I never give her a prescription but only a two-month supply of the pill that is best suited for her, along with instructions to return as she nears the end of the second packet of pills. If she wants to continue on the pill, she has to come back. Then I again take her blood pressure and examine her breasts; I may repeat lab studies, including blood sugar, lipids, and liver profile. The patient and I review her mental and physical state and decide whether to continue her medication. If she has become depressed (possibly because of pill-related abnormalities in B_6 metabolism), I make sure her supplemental vitamins contain B_6. We also might try a different pill or change to a different form of contraception. The patient, thereafter, will return for a physical examination and appropriate laboratory blood work every six months while she is on the pill.

There are women who should never take the pill because they have an increased risk of serious side effects. If you have at any time in your life had any of the following conditions, you should *not* use an oral contraceptive.[14]

1. heart attack or stroke
2. blood clots in the legs or lungs

3. angina pectoris (pain in the chest associated with a heart condition)
4. cancer of the breast or sex organs, or suspected cancer of these areas
5. unusual vaginal bleeding that has not been diagnosed
6. liver disease or seriously impaired liver function
7. confirmed or suspected pregnancy (if you are already on the pill, stop taking it)

Several other situations also preclude use of the pill:

If you have irregular periods—that is, if you occasionally skip a month or two—or if you have been having your periods for less than two years, you should not use the pill. In either case, if you do, you may have difficulty becoming pregnant when you are ready to have a child, or you may not menstruate when you discontinue the pill.

If you smoke, think twice before deciding to take the pill. Cigarette smoking increases the risk of serious side effects associated with oral contraceptives. If you don't know which one to give up, forgo your cigarettes and take the pill. The pill is safer than cigarettes, and its advantages are more fun. Smoking alone increases the risk of many circulatory disease for women, regardless of their contraceptive method. Smoking and oral contraceptives combined produce an effect greater than the sum of their individual effects. Heart attack and hemorrhagic stroke, particularly subarachnoid (brain) hemorrhage, show this effect most clearly.

In addition to the indications that absolutely rule out the pill, there are other conditions that might be aggravated by them. If you have one or more of them, your physician should closely monitor you while you are taking the pill. If possible, I would recommend that you consider an alternate method, because the benefits of the pill if you have one of these conditions are not worth the risk:

1. a family history of breast cancer
2. breast nodules, fibrocystic breast disease, abnormal mammogram

3. diabetes
4. high blood pressure
5. high cholesterol or triglyceride level
6. cigarette smoking
7. migraine headaches
8. heart, kidney, or liver disease
9. epilepsy
10. mental depression
11. fibroid tumors of the uterus
12. gall bladder disease
13. menstrual periods that are grossly irregular

Women over 35 who have conditions predisposing them to circulatory-system disease, such as obesity, hypertension, high cholesterol level, diabetes, and, most important, smoking, are the group at greatest risk.

Despite the hazards, oral contraceptives remain the most popular contraceptive choice of younger women in the United States. Fortunately, the trend has been away from pills with high doses of hormones to pills that contain 50 micrograms or less of estrogen; yet oral contraceptives with more than 80 micrograms of estrogen still constitute more than 25 percent of sales. I am appalled by the number of patients coming into my practice who are taking high-dose pills. I immediately transfer these women to lower-dose pills, but many doctors seem to keep on renewing their old prescriptions without regard to the fact that the newer, lower-dose pills are safer.

Most young women ask for the pill, and it is best suited to this age group. If there are no major contraindications, and if your menstrual periods are regular (regular means occurring once every three to six weeks), and if after considering all the alternatives, the pill is what you want, you should get it. See your doctor within two to three months after starting on the pill to be sure that your blood pressure is not rising and that any symptoms that could be danger signs are thoroughly investigated. Thereafter, you should return for an examination and blood tests every six to twelve months; and because vitamin deficiencies develop in all women who are on the pill, you should take a multiple vitamin (including B_6) with minerals daily.

The advantages of oral contraceptives are:

1. They are 99 percent effective if each and every pill is taken. (If pills are forgotten, the percentage decreases.)
2. They decrease menstrual flow and pain.
3. They do not interfere with spontaneity or sensation during intercourse.

The disadvantages are:

1. They may cause serious side effects, which can even be fatal.
2. They shut off the woman's entire reproductive-hormone system.
3. All the long-term effects are not yet known.
4. They do not protect against sexually transmitted disease.
5. They require close medical supervision.
6. Users can easily forget to take them.
7. They can cause mental depression in some users.
8. Supplemental vitamins should be taken along with them.

STERILIZATION PROCEDURES

Sterilization is a surgical procedure that provides permanent contraception. It should be considered nonreversible and is extremely effective for anyone who has decided not to have children ever, or ever again. Either the female or the male partner can be sterilized. When performed on the female (tubal ligation), the operation is considered major surgery. As in any other major surgical procedure, there are associated complications as well as some risk of dying. The procedure is infinitely simpler and safer when performed on the male (vasectomy).

Tubal Ligation

This is accomplished by cutting, tying, burning, clipping, or otherwise blocking the fallopian tubes so that the egg produced in the ovary cannot pass to the uterus. The obstruction of the tubes prevents the sperm from coming into contact with the egg; and because the egg and the sperm are prevented from meeting, fertilization cannot take place. The fallopian tubes, lying deep in the abdominal cavity, must first be exposed by the surgeon; and though various techniques can be used to expose the tubes, all of them require that the abdomen be opened.

Four types of tubal ligation are performed: laparotomy, laparoscopy, vaginal tube ligation, and postpartum tubal ligation; the type you receive probably will depend on your doctor. The procedures are not exactly the same, and the size and location of the surgical scar, as well as the required recuperation period, can vary considerably. You should have the opportunity to select the procedure you want, unless there is a medical reason why it is not right for you. If you decide on sterilization, make sure that both you and your surgeon know what type you want. If your doctor doesn't agree to perform that type or has had very little experience with it, find another doctor.

LAPAROTOMY In this oldest sterilization procedure, the surgeon makes a three- to five-inch incision in the abdomen, sufficient to expose the fallopian tubes. He then either removes a section from each tube and ties the ends with surgical thread, or he seals them with electric cautery, bands, or clips. The method the surgeon uses to seal the fallopian tubes is important, in terms of both safety and effectiveness. The most common method is the Pomeroy technique: the surgeon lifts each tube to create a loop, ties the base of the loop firmly together with suture, and cuts off the top of the loop. In about a week, the suture is absorbed and the two scarred ends of the tube pull apart, leaving a gap between them.

Some surgeons do variations of this procedure by using

a different suture material or by blocking the fimbria (the fingers of the fallopian tube that receive the egg from the ovary). Once the tubes are blocked, the incision is closed with stitches.

Laparotomy usually requires a general anesthetic and takes about thirty minutes. Patients usually spend four days in the hospital and often do not feel like their former selves again for six weeks. Of all the sterilization procedures, this one has the highest rate of failure (1 to 3 percent pregnancy), costs more, and has the highest rate of complications. Still, it is the procedure of choice when there has been a history of complicated abdominal surgery with adhesions resulting from infection—for example, from a ruptured appendix.

MINILAPAROTOMY   This simplication of the laparotomy is easier and quicker to perform. An instrument is inserted into the uterus through the cervix and is used to push the uterus up against the abdominal wall. The surgeon then makes a small (about one inch) incision in the skin above the uterus, exposing the fallopian tubes. (Sometimes the surgeon may use a retractor, which operates somewhat like a small speculum, to help him locate the tubes.) He ties or severs the tubes and closes the incision. This procedure takes twenty to thirty minutes. It can be done under local anesthesia, but very often a general anesthetic is used. In many countries, the patient goes home from the hospital the same day, but in the United States, women remain in the hospital for a couple more days. It takes about two weeks at home before the patient feels normal again.

LAPAROSCOPY   This technique is commonly called Band-Aid surgery, because the incision required is so small (about half an inch) that it can be closed and covered by an adhesive strip.

The laparoscope is a long tube that is slightly thicker than a pencil, which is inserted into the abdomen. Laparoscopy has become very popular during the last decade because of the development of fiberoptics, a system that permits cold light to be transported through the instrument to illuminate the operative field inside the abdomen. The laparoscope functions like a hollow flashlight, enabling the surgeon to see the internal organs and to insert operating tools through the hollow bore of the instrument.

The surgeon first makes a small incision near the navel. A long, thin needle is inserted into the abdominal cavity through the incision, and about 2 liters of an inert, harmless gas (carbon dioxide or nitrous oxide) are pumped through the needle to inflate the abdomen. The gas helps prevent surgical accidents by pushing the intestines away from the uterus and the tubes. The laparoscope is then inserted through the incision, and the fallopian tubes are individually isolated and sealed. (Some surgeons make a second small incision at the pubic hairline to insert the operating instruments.)

The most common method employed during laparoscopy is cauterization, using electricity. The cautery, a coagulation forceps, is passed through the laparoscope to grasp the tube; then current is applied in short bursts to burn and seal it. Recently, because of the dangers of cautery, clips and rings that can pass through the laparoscope are often being used. The silastic ring (or falope ring), for example, can be slipped over a tubal loop, which the surgeon forms in the same manner as in the Pomeroy technique. The new Hulka clip simply clips the tube closed. In theory, these procedures have the advantage of being easily reversible, because no portion of the fallopian tube is removed or severely damaged, as it is with cautery; but since these new techniques are not as well documented as cautery, it is possible that they may be slightly less effective in preventing pregnancy.

After the tubes are sealed, the instruments are withdrawn, the gas is released, the incision is closed with one stitch, and the Band-Aid is applied. The procedure takes about thirty minutes and is usually done under general anesthesia. The hospital stay usually lasts one day, and the patient is back to normal in two or three days. Many patients, however, complain about pain; it usually eases after twenty-four hours, but some women report discomfort for one or two weeks.

VAGINAL TUBAL LIGATION   In this procedure, the surgeon exposes the fallopian tubes by making his incision deep in the vagina in order to open the abdominal cavity. He may use a different instrument, called a culdoscope, which also has a light source, to visualize the tubes. The operation takes about thirty minutes, and the hospital stay usually is one day. After two or three more days, the patient feels normal but should not have intercourse for about a month to allow the incision in the vagina to heal. This procedure, which has more potential for infection (because the doctor is operating through an incision in the nonsterile vagina) and more bleeding, is declining in popularity.

POSTPARTUM TUBAL LIGATION   A tubal ligation can be performed anytime, including right after childbirth, while the woman is still in the hospital, the uterus is still enlarged, and the fallopian tubes are much easier to locate.

The surgeon makes a one- to two-inch incision below the navel, isolating and sealing the tubes. It takes about thirty minutes. An additional day or two may be added to the hospital stay, but the patient usually feels back to normal in about the same time it would take to recover from the childbirth alone.

Many doctors feel that the postpartum period is an ideal time for a woman to have a tubal ligation. If she already has several children, is lying on the table, and has left her signed permission on file, the woman's physician is likely to feel that the time is perfect for the procedure. Surgery at this time, however, can be technically more difficult and dangerous because of the greater size of the pelvic organs and their greater vascularity. Increased blood flow through the enlarged blood vessels, for example, increases the danger of hemorrhage. And should anything happen to the patient's newborn baby, she may regret her decision for immediate tubal ligation.

* * *

No matter which of the techniques described is used, its purpose is to isolate the fallopian tubes so that they can be sealed. All the procedures seem simple and safe enough, but things do not always go well.

In performing any of these procedures, the surgeon, working through a small opening, is trying to isolate and seal a couple of tiny tubes that he must first find and accurately identify. Sometimes he thinks he has the proper tube when in reality he may have sealed a ureter, blocking the flow of urine into the bladder, causing very serious problems and requiring immediate surgery to reverse the error. With his instruments, the surgeon also might perforate the bowel or a blood vessel in the abdomen. With the cautery, he might inadvertently burn the intestine, resulting in serious infectious complications. The heat from the cautery may spread to the adjacent tissue and cause destruction of or decrease in the nearby blood supply to the ovary. Less disastrous slips or misidentifications might result in the cautery or clipping of one of the supporting ligaments of the uterus. If this error goes unnoticed, a fallopian tube is left open and the woman is not protected from pregnancy.

The complication rate for tubal ligation varies between 3 and 5 percent, depending on the procedure and the surgeon. Some of the complications, such as a blood clot in the lung, bleeding from a damaged blood vessel, and cardiac arrest, can be fatal. While these are rare, as many as seventy-five women die each year as a direct result of tubal ligation.[15] This number includes the mortality risk from anesthesia when a general anesthetic is used.

When it is properly performed, of course, the tubal ligation should guarantee 100 percent effective birth control, but the actual effectiveness is somewhat less than 100 percent because the seal may not completely block the tube or may be applied to the wrong tube. Or the tube may repair itself later on. Should pregnancy occur, there is an increased possibility of tubal pregnancy.

In addition, the scientific literature is currently reporting that women who have undergone tubal sterilization, especially with cautery technique, subsequently have higher hysterectomy rates. By destroying tissue and vessels, the tubal surgery interferes with the blood supply of the ovary. A blood-deprived ovary may no longer function perfectly; its hormonal output may be decreased, making ovulation irregular. The result is an abnormal pattern of uterine bleeding that becomes the basis for the increased rates of hysterectomy.

Current researchers are trying to find ways of blocking the tubes that do not require surgical penetration of the abdomen or the vagina. A new procedure that shows promise uses an instrument called a hysteroscope. Similar to the laparoscope, it is inserted into the uterus through the small opening in the cervix (the os) instead of through an incision in the abdomen. Once the hysteroscope is inside the uterus, the surgeon can locate the two openings where the fallopian tubes attach to the uterus and seal them by inserting a plug, injecting a silicone-rubber sealant, or injecting a scarring agent.

Sterilization by tubal ligation should be considered only when any future pregnancy would be a catastrophe, because I think that the risks of tubal ligation outweigh its possible benefits. The younger woman, who receives the benefit of a long period of contraception, risks future years of poor ovarian function. The older woman receives less contraceptive time benefit from sterilization. Also, as women mature, they become less fertile. As she approaches menopause, using a foam or a diaphragm or an IUD is far less bothersome than the complications of a tubal ligation might be.

If you feel you have no viable option, however, and have made up your mind to undergo sterilization, I favor laparoscopy with the use of the falope ring. Avoid cautery if possible. A recent improvement in the cautery, however, permits more careful control of the electrical current, decreasing the risk of inadvertent burns, so if your surgeon intends to use cautery, ask if he is using this newer "bipolar cautery" technique.

Laparoscopy became a commonly taught procedure in the late 1960s and has been an important part of the training of the obstetrician/gynecologist. If your gynecologist is older, he may well have learned the technique in postgraduate courses, which tend to be fairly short and less thorough than the training a surgeon receives during residency. Therefore, it might be advisable to choose a doctor who received his training after the procedures became part of the training program, a doctor who teaches the procedure to residents, or a doctor who has done at least two hundred procedures.

Should you choose tubal ligation, however, you must have a Pap test and a pelvic examination first. If, by some misfortune, you turn out to have cancer of the cervix, huge fibroids, or abnormal bleeding due to uterine cancer, it would make little sense to have a tubal ligation when hysterectomy might well be the better choice.

On a more personal note, because the procedure usually is irreversible, elect tubal ligation only when your life is fairly stable. Most of the requests to have tubal surgery reversed come from women who underwent tubal ligation just after they got divorced, then remarried, and now want a child.

To sum up the advantages of tubal ligation:

1. It is a one-time procedure with a one-time cost.
2. It is nearly 100 percent effective.
3. It does not interfere with spontaneity during intercourse.

The disadvantages are:

1. It is permanent and should be considered irreversible. Even when reversals can be made, subsequent pregnancy rates are poor.
2. It may interfere with the blood supply of the ovaries and lead to abnormal hormonal production, lack of ovulation, unusual bleeding patterns, and a need for later surgery, including hysterectomy.
3. The full implications of the procedures won't be known for at least another decade.

4. The surgery may have serious complications such as hemorrhage, peritonitis from bowel burns, infection of the wound and so on. Even without complications, it causes postoperative pain.
5. Should the procedure fail and pregnancy occur, there is an increased risk of tubal pregnancy.

Vasectomy

For the woman considering sterilization, I recommend that her husband have a vasectomy instead. I am amazed at the number of women who choose to undergo this operation because they do not want to ask their husbands to have surgery. They are willing to risk their lives so that their husbands will not have a moment's discomfort. Some of these women have overwhelming maternal concern for their spouses or feel terribly beholden to them. Others feel that they are stronger and that their husbands will not be able to endure even a minor operative procedure. Some fear that their husbands may wander, while others fear that the surgery will permanently damage their sexual ability. However, no woman should elect to be sterilized without first exploring the possibility of a vasectomy with her husband.

Vasectomy is a 99-percent effective procedure. It is much simpler and safer than any of the sterilization procedures available for women, because the male sex organs, being located outside the body, are easily accessible. Consequently, the surgery required to expose the vas deferens of the male is much less serious than the abdominal surgery needed to expose a woman's fallopian tubes.

The vas deferens is a tube that transports sperm from the testicle, where it is manufactured, to the prostate gland, where it is added to the ejaculate. Just as there are two fallopian tubes in women (one for each ovary), there are two vas deferens in men (one for each testicle). In performing a vasectomy, the surgeon makes a small slit in the skin of the scrotum (the skin sac that holds the testicles) to expose the vas. Then, the vas is cut, tied, clamped, or otherwise obstructed so that sperm can no longer pass. This procedure is exactly analogous to a female sterilization during which the fallopian tubes are obstructed so that the egg cannot pass on to the uterus.

A vasectomy takes about twenty minutes and is usually performed in the physician's office under a local, dental-type anesthetic that is injected into the skin of the scrotum at the site of each of the two incisions. The cost is about $200.

There has never been a vasectomy-associated death in the United States. Minor complications such as pain, swelling, or occasional infection of the incision site may occur, but these result in only minor discomfort for a few days. Ninety-five percent of the men who have had vasectomies do not hesitate to recommend it to other men. Consequently, the popularity of vasectomy has been on the upswing for the last decade; as many as 750,000 men in the United States now elect it each year. Five percent of the men who have had vasectomies, however, have had a difficult psychological adjustment to it, which often manifests itself in impotency. For this reason, no male should ever allow himself to be talked into a vasectomy. The procedure must be thought of as irreversible, although occasionally it may be successfully undone. The decision for vasectomy should be made only if the male is absolutely certain that he does not want to father any more children, regardless of any future circumstance.

There are many misconceptions about vasectomy, perhaps resulting from the early history of the procedure. About fifty years ago, it was used primarily to sterilize criminals, mental defectives, and those with hereditary diseases. This disreputable history may contribute to the psychological distress that some men—the unhappy 5 percent—experience following vasectomy. Nevertheless, vasectomy is *not* castration, nor does it in any way interfere with normal male function during intercourse. In fact, many men report an increase in their sexuality following vasectomy. The only thing missing is about one drop of fluid in the ejaculate, which would have contained millions of sperm. Neither partner can notice its absence, nor can anyone in any way tell that the male has had a vasectomy.

After vasectomy, the sperm that continue to be manufactured are absorbed by the body; and men who have had a vasectomy may develop antibodies to sperm. This phenomenon has never resulted in any widespread symptoms of adverse health in men, but some researchers warn of vague possible effects on body organs. Along that same line, a researcher has noted that vasectomy caused an increase in cholesterol in ten monkeys.[16] (The same ten monkeys are referred to again and again in the medical literature.) However, a recent Boston study of 10,000 vasectomized men followed for a period of ten years showed no increase in heart attack rates compared with men who had not had the surgery.

I have always been fascinated by the fact that the research establishment warns about a theoretical risk to men, while it accepts a proven danger to women as inevitable. We know of the many adverse effects of "the pill"—including death—and we know that women die every year during sterilization surgery. Yet these deaths are minimized by the male-dominated medical profession. Female sterilization is promoted as "Band-Aid" surgery, even though it is major surgery that is usually performed in a hospital under full anesthesia.

On the other hand, vasectomy, which has no death rate at all, no serious complications, and is simply a minor, doctor's-office procedure—after which the patient gets up and walks home—is found by researchers to have *theoretical* risks that must be taken seriously. To me, this attitude epitomizes the sexism of medicine. If a couple decides on a permanent method of sterilization, it makes sense that the partner at least risk should have the procedure. When one compares the risks of tubal ligation to the risks of vasectomy, there can be no question as to the safest procedure. Every time a man turns down a vasectomy to avoid a theoretical risk, is partner becomes subject to a tubal ligation that carries a very definite risk. For those couples seeking a permanent method of contraception, then, vasectomy is the most reasonable solution.

NEW DEVELOPMENT—THE CERVICAL CAP

With a little luck, a new contraceptive option for women—the cervical cap—may be on the market in a few years. Tests are currently in progress to determine the effectiveness of the caps, pregnancy rates, patient acceptance, and long-term problems requiring changes in technique or materials.

The cervical cap is a barrier device that fits over the cervix and prevents sperm from entering the uterus. It functions something like a diaphragm, but it is only one-third to one-half as big—about 30 millimeters in diameter—because it is designed to cover only the cervix and not (like the diaphragm) part of the vagina as well. And while the diaphragm is held in place by the pressure of its flexible rim against the vaginal wall, the custom-fit cervical cap stays put because it fits so exactly.

Cervical caps that looked like tiny diaphragms were sold many years ago. They had to be placed on the cervix and could be left in place for a day or so, but they had to be removed prior to menses. It took a very adept woman to insert one correctly, and even so, these old rubber caps often became dislodged during intercourse. They never achieved a high degree of reliability.

At least two models are currently under investigation. Both feature a valve which allows menstrual fluid or mucus to flow from the uterus into the vagina but blocks sperm from entering the uterus. One of these caps was designed by a gynecologist in association with a dentist.[17] Working on the principle that the cap would be most likely to remain in position if it could be made to fit the cervix exactly, they made precise molds of the cervix, much like those a dentist makes of the gums in order to fit a denture. Once an impression of the cervix is taken, a plaster cast is made; the cap is fabricated on the plaster mold and then positioned on the cervix by the doctor. The entire process takes about half an hour. Since it is equipped with a one-way valve, the device can be left in place for from several months to a couple of years.

The other cap currently under investigation is not custommade but comes in several sizes that closely approximate varying cervical anatomies.

One of the complaints often cited in the scientific literature about barrier devices is that they become malodorous, especially if they are worn for more than twenty-four hours. The cause is similar to the cause of denture odor. If the device does not fit well, there are places where mucus can accumulate in stagnant pools; as it is broken down by microbial action, unpleasant odors are produced. If the device fits exactly, however, mucus flows smoothly underneath it, and the constant flow of mucus cleans the device.

The longest continuously worn custom cap was in place for twenty-two months without cervical irritation, odor, or any other detectable adverse effects.[18] Moreover, because the cap is placed over the cervix and not inside the uterus, like the IUD, its placement is painless and less likely to result in complications. Experimentation with this promising device continues, and if it is successful, women will be able to choose this method from the growing list of available contraceptive procedures.

There are also caps without valves that are currently available from some of the women's health centers and, rarely, from physicians. Because of the need for exact fit and detailed, consuming explanations about placement, caps have not been readily accepted by the medical community. I feel that because of the sudden emergence of Toxic Shock Syndrome (TSS), any device placed in the vagina for an extended period of time must be well researched to rule out the possibility of adverse effects. Until long-term, scientifically controlled studies have confirmed the safety of such devices, I must regard all of them as experimental.

* * *

From time to time stories have appeared in the press endorsing electronic, oral temperature-taking devices that can be used to determine the time of ovulation. Such a device is now being tested in England by the British Medical Research Council in family-planning clinics.

CONTRACEPTION COSTS

Method	Approximate Annual Costs (Assuming 100 sex acts per year)
Modified abstinence (Rhythm—calendar/ temperature)	None
Coitus interruptus	None
Spermicides (Jelly, cream, foam, suppository)	$25–40
Diaphragm and spermicide	$45–65 (plus doctor's office fee)
Condom	$50–125
IUD—nonmedicated	$35–75 "amortized" over 5 years = $7–15/year
IUD—copper	$50–100 "amortized" over 3 years = $17–33/year
IUD—progesterone	$50–100/year
Oral contraceptives	$75 (plus doctor's office fee)
Menstrual regulation	$90–150 (x procedures/year)
Abortion (first trimester)	$150–300 (x procedures/year)
Sterilization, male	$175–300 "amortized" over 10 years = $17–30/year
Sterilization, female	$400–850 "amortized" over 10 years =$40–85/year

CONTRACEPTIVE EFFECTIVENESS

Method	Percentage of Approximate Effectiveness
Combined oral contraceptive	98–99
Condom combined with spermicide (foam)	98–99
Intrauterine contraceptive	95–98
Diaphragm and spermicide	90–94
Condom	90–95
Spermicide	88–94
Rhythm—calendar	79
Douching	60
Chance	15
Male sterilization	99+
Female sterilization	99+

After the device has been tested and made available to the public, it will make birth control less of a mystery. For couples who use no other method of birth control, the device will indicate those times when it is necessary to abstain from sex. For couples who use mechanical contraceptives, the device will indicate those times when it is safe to have sex without using contraceptive devices.

Given all the options, how do you decide which method of contraception is best for you? Many factors should influence your choice, and only you can weigh them all. Consider your age, the number of childbearing years ahead of you, and your desire (or lack of desire) to have children at some later date. Younger women need the protection from cervical cancer provided by the condom, while women over 35 can't risk the pill. Consider your sexual and social habits. If you have a number of partners or frequently meet new partners, you need condom and foam protection from venereal disease. And to be on the safe side, remember: you know whom you are sleeping with, but you don't know whom he is sleeping with. If you have sexual relations infrequently, you don't need the constant protection of the

pill or an IUD. Of course, if your religion forbids contraceptive devices, you do not have access to a physician, or
you cannot afford some of the more expensive methods
(and the necessary follow-up medical care), then your choices
are considerably narrowed.

The final choice will be a personal one, but some recommendations apply to women in all age groups. Be aware
of the problem of venereal disease, and protect yourself,
especially at the start of a new relationship. Be aware of
the problems that accompany tubal ligation, and make that
decision carefully. Be honest with yourself. If you lack the
discipline to take time out in the heat of passion to get
that diaphragm or foam out of the drawer, choose another
method of birth control now, before it's too late. On the
other hand, if you are using contraception to space pregnancies rather than to prevent them and would not greatly
mind becoming pregnant, even if it is not the most convenient time, then neglecting to use your foam or diaphragm
occasionally is no disaster.

Learn about the various methods of contraception and
experiment with them; otherwise you might miss one that
could be especially good for you. If you are in a stable
relationship, sometimes it is nice to share the responsibility
for birth control. For example, right after your period, you
might use only foam. In mid-cycle, during your fertile time,
condom and foam combined would be a good method; and
then before your period, he could use condoms. Or you
might use just foam after your period and a diaphragm for
another part of your cycle. If you elect to use an IUD, add
foam in the middle of the month, especially if you are using
a smaller-size nonmedicated device. Be willing to change
as your social circumstances change; remember that only
sterilization is forever.

Above all, remember that although women still bear the
major responsibility for birth control, the good news is that
more and more options are available. The choice is up to
you.

CHAPTER 4

No More Radical
Mastectomies

Breast cancer is hardly a cheerful topic, even though 93 percent of women will never get it. But the more you know about breast cancer and all the latest techniques of detection, the better able you will be to defend yourself against it. Early detection is the real key to survival in breast cancer. The more prompt the diagnosis, the better the survival statistics. And 90 percent of all breast cancer is first detected by the patient.

Unfortunately, most women refuse to think about it at all. They block it out of their minds and try to pretend it doesn't exist, at least not for them. It is often not the possibility of death that conjures up awful images for them but the aftermath of surgery and its mutilation. Yet the good news about breast cancer is that its victims need *not* be mutilated. Radical mastectomy—the old, disfiguring operation—is no longer necessary.

For most women, having breasts is synonymous with being female. As little girls, we saw our developing breasts as the first sign that we were becoming women. As women, we realized that our breasts are more than mere symbols of being female; they are organs of sexual pleasure. They are comparable in men not to the male breasts but to the testicles. Like the testes, breasts are not directly involved in the sex act, but they carry intense feelings and sensations and they are essential to sexual identity. If a man had to have one or both of his testes removed, he could pad out his underwear with cotton, just as mastectomy victims pad their flattened chests, but he would always be hesitant to show himself to his partner; he would always worry about the fit and draping of his trousers. Would it show? Would anyone see that he had become "less" than a man?

That's how women feel. Surgeons try to comfort their patients by explaining that a woman is a woman whether she has one breast or two or none, and that the important thing is to save her life. A woman awaiting surgery can know that such reasoning is sound, but deep down, on an emotional level, she knows that her life will never be the same again.

And indeed it may not be. Studies show that women who undergo radical mastectomies often experience a major change—usually a decline—in their sex lives. About one-third may stop having sexual relations altogether.[1] In a majority of reported cases, husbands of radical-mastectomy victims have not seen their wives unclothed even two years after the operation.

On the brighter side, women who undergo lesser procedures, which leave the breast intact, seem to maintain their sexual identity and to carry on a normal sex life.

Today breast-cancer care is not as traumatic as it was even five years ago. Then there was no alternative to the radical, mutilating surgery that removed not only the breast but the underlying muscle wall and the underarm lymph glands as well; but doctors are now using various treatments—including techniques such as radiation alone and combined with minimal surgical techniques (lumpectomy)—which leave the breast intact. These techniques have five-year survival rates *equal* to the more radical surgical procedures in women with early breast cancer. A panel of cancer specialists convened by the National Cancer Institute in 1979 agreed that the century-old radical procedure should no longer be used in treatment of early breast cancer.[2] Clearly, then, there is good news to talk about: less surgery and less radical surgery.

Perhaps, knowing these facts, we can overcome the terrible dread of mutilation that has contributed to the awful survival rates for breast cancer in this country. As things stand now, even well-educated women who are in every other way clever, intelligent, and reasonable, childishly refuse even to examine their own bodies. Sophisticated women find lumps yet refuse to go to their doctors to have them checked. Ninety-three to 97 percent of women with diagnosed breast cancer who do *not* get treatment die within ten years of the discovery of the disease. Sadly, women must share part of the blame for these grim breast-cancer statistics.

A woman is most likely to come to her physician because she noticed something unusual about her breast: a lump, swelling, nipple discharge, or pain. But since most women don't do systematic breast self-examination, they only find their tumors when they are large and obvious. Tumors may grow to be two or three centimeters before the average woman notices anything unusual. By the time the tumor reaches that size, it has already been there for more than two years, perhaps even five or more, and chances are that her cancer is no longer localized. Almost one-half of all breast cancers occur in women 45 to 65 years old; and in only 43 percent of these cases is cancer diagnosed while it is still localized. Consequently, the overall survival rate for this group is only 60 percent.

But there is little excuse for such a gloomy figure. There are many opportunities to find that lump earlier—*much, much earlier*. Breast self-examination, performed religiously every month, will discover tumors while they are still small and provide an 80 percent survival rate at five years. When you consider that the survival rates apply only to the 7 percent of women who will ever get breast cancer, the figures are really pretty good. Other new screening techniques, which I'll discuss later, make those figures even better.

BREAST SELF-EXAMINATION

In order to be effective, Breast Self-Examination (BSE) must become a habit. You should examine your breasts once a month, immediately after your period has ended. If you do it before your period, you probably will scare yourself to death. Breasts tend to be extra tender and lumpy for a week or so before the onset of flow. After menses, your breasts will be somewhat softer, and most of the bumpiness will have disappeared, making the examination less confusing. Doctors themselves get confused by the lumps and bumps that occur premenstrually and often ask women to return after menstruation.

Most women attempting BSE for the first time complain that they don't know which lumps are important and which are not. While some women have nearly perfectly smooth breast tissue that follows an easy and straightforward examination, most women are not so fortunate. Whenever I instruct a patient in BSE, I point out the woman's most obvious bumps and show her how to recognize the insignificant ones: they move easily and are very much like many of the other, smaller lumps in her breast. I alert her to the fact that they may become firm premenstrually. Once my patient actually feels these areas under my supervision, she can then do her own examination at home without any trouble. I ask her to reexamine her breasts when she gets home that very day to become familiar with her normal anatomy, bumpy or not. Then if a new lump appears, she will recognize it.

Although most women know about BSE, only a few (18 percent) practice it. Statistics show that most women do not do BSE because they don't feel confident that they can distinguish a lump from normal breast tissue. But the only way to learn is to practice. Once a woman is thoroughly acquainted with her own breast anatomy, she may be a better diagnostician than her doctor, who examines many women and cannot possibly remember every detail. It is possible that he might miss some nuance that the patient would be aware of if she performed a diligent monthly breast assessment.

So it is up to you to learn BSE. Ask your physician to teach you. Or if you begin at home on your own, do not be ashamed to ask your doctor questions about areas you may be concerned about. If the physician examines you but will not take the time to show you how to do BSE, then examine your breasts after you have returned home and assume that all you feel is normal breast tissue. Use this examination as a baseline for your future self-examination. And definitely consider changing your doctor.

The first step in BSE is to look in the mirror and become familiar with the shape and outline of your breasts. Look for any lumps or thickening of the skin that you can see. Note the position of your nipples, observe whether either seems to be pulled to the left, right, or out of its normal position, possibly by a tumor underneath it. Is one nipple newly inverted, or is there a noticeable scaling or secretion? As you look into the mirror with your arms by your sides, raise your arms over your head and continue to look at your breasts. Push your hands together over your head, continue looking, and then put your hands on your hips and press down on them. This tenses your chest muscles and gives a slightly different perspective to your breasts. Now lie on your bed. If your breasts are full, place a flat pillow or a folded towel under your left shoulder. Raise your left arm over your head and rest it comfortably back on the bed. Using the fleshy part of your fingertips but not the very tips, begin making small, circular motions with your right hand. Begin at the colored edge of the nipple. From there, as if your breast were a clock, feel out along the entire breast at twelve o'clock, one o'clock, two o'clock, and so on, until you have systematically felt the entire breast. In the portion of the breast near your underarm, feel all the way to where your armpit begins. In the lower portion of your breast, you should find a ridge of firm tissue. This is part of the natural supporting tissue of the breast and always makes the underneath portion of the breast feel firmer. Finally, feel up into your armpit. Some women have noticeable lymph nodes there,* while others do not. If you find a node, it should move freely, feel soft, and not be tender. When you are finished, shift the pillow to your right side and repeat the whole process. At the end of the procedure, squeeze your nipples gently to see if any secretion or blood is present.

If you find a lump, dimple, discharge, or any other change in the appearance or feel of your breasts since your last examination, see your doctor—immediately. Although 80 percent of breast lumps and other changes are benign and not cancerous, it's not worth taking a chance, ever.

BSE is simple, inexpensive, and noninvasive; but some doctors are not convinced that it is worth the effort. A doctor stated in the *New England Journal of Medicine:* "It is a common experience that patients have a certain fear, dislike or dread of BSE, and that they do not trust themselves."[3] One patient asked him if a group of male physicians would be willing to drop their Levi's and BVDs in front of a mirror once a month and examine both testicles carefully, looking for tumors. He thought that the woman had made a good point and that self-examination is of too intimate a nature and only arouses thoughts of cancer and death. I disagree. Why shouldn't every male learn to examine his testicles for early cancer? Neither men nor women should be so shy and fearful about their anatomy. Breast self-examination should be taught in every high school so that it can become a habit of good health rather than a desperate measure.

BREAST CHANGES FROM ADOLESCENCE TO MATURITY

As breasts develop, grow, and mature, many different lumps, masses, and symptoms may appear. When you practice BSE, you should be aware of what you are likely to find at different stages in your life.

*Small, mobile glands in the armpit, lymph nodes produce lymphocytes— white blood cells—which fight infection.

The normal breast is composed of fatty areas and glands that produce milk. Some breasts contain more fat, while others, especially the firmer breasts of young women, have more gland than fat. The gland tissue tends to be more lumpy, while fat is softer and smooth. Most of the glandular tissue is found in the lateral upper portion of the breast, near the underarm area; and it is in that upper outer quadrant of the breast that most breast cancers (60 percent) arise. (When you feel this portion of the breast during BSE, if it contains a large amount of breast glands, the area will just slide back and forth over your chest wall.)

Between the ages of 7 and 10, a boy or girl may have a firm, buttonlike, flat-topped bump lying directly beneath his or her nipple. Often it may appear only in one breast. This solid little button of tissue is actually the potential gland of the breast, just ready to bloom. Many a child has appeared in the doctor's office accompanied by a distraught mother who has been taught that all breast lumps are cancer. On rare occasions, these breast buds have been biopsied (partially removed for microscopic examination) or even completely removed. These procedures lead to distortion or the complete absence of breast development. Breast cancer in the adolescent and the woman under 30 is rare. There are only thirteen cases in the medical literature on children between the ages of 6 and 15, and only 1 percent of breast cancers occur in women under 30.[4]

FIBROADENOMAS

Breast tumors called fibroadenomas are common at all ages but occur most often in young women from menarche to age 35. They are nontender, firm, smooth, and rubbery, and move about as you push them from side to side. They are not adherent to the skin overlying them or the tissue below them. Often you will find several. These tumors, like cysts, are firm because they are composed of a fibrous capsule which compresses the soft tissue inside. Some doctors will simply monitor them, especially in a very young teenager.

Because they can be confused with more serious growths, they are often removed using dental-type local anesthesia in the over-20-year-old group.

CYSTS

The most common benign breast problem is the cyst. Perhaps 30 percent of women have them. If there is a lump that always seems to swell and become tender before your menses and then become smaller and less tender afterward, you probably have found a cyst. Fluctuations in size are rare in other benign or malignant tumors of the breast. Cystic breast disease, also known as fibrocystic disease or chronic cystic mastitis, is the source of much concern in the 30–40 age group, for it is often confused with malignancy. Cysts are most usually found in this age group, though they may occur at any time in a woman's reproductive life. However, after a woman is a year or two into menopause, breast cysts rarely occur.

A cyst feels like a movable marble within the tissue of the breast. If there are multiple small cysts, however, the entire area may not be as freely movable as when there are only single cysts. Cysts may be tender or painful, depending on their number, size, location, and rate of enlargement. They may be firm to hard, because they contain fluid that is tightly compressed within the fibrous capsule, somewhat like a balloon filled to capacity with water. Before your menses, because of the increased fluid, these cysts fill and become bigger and, therefore, harder. Not only will the lump appear hard and even painful, but it may suddenly appear where last week you could detect nothing. If you can survive the week (mentally) until after your flow has stopped, you will find that the cyst either has disappeared or has gotten much smaller and softer. The cyst is still there, of course, but like a deflated balloon it no longer has structure or volume.

Women who have breast cysts should be seen for a breast check more frequently than women who don't—at least twice a year—for two reasons. First, patients who have cystic disease are three to four times more likely to develop breast cancer[5] (although the actual presence of a cancer in a noticeable cyst is extremely rare; 99.5 percent of the time, there is no cancer within the cyst itself[6]). The second reason is the increased risk that arises from the possibility of a malignancy developing within the breast, which cannot be differentiated from all of the surrounding cysts.

Other Benign Findings

There are other benign diseases of the breast in the 30–40 age group, including some types of overgrowth of the milk ducts, known as intraductal papillomas; or overgrowth of milk ducts and surrounding connective tissue, known as sclerosing adenosis. They add to the confusion when trying to decide if a breast contains a tumor that needs to be biopsied or just watched. Other, rarer problems, such as fat necrosis, may occur if the breast is injured, a not unusual occurrence. The injured fat becomes irritated, and bleeding may occur in the area after injury. This damage results in a stony, hard area, and in the healing process, the overlying skin retracts as it would in an advanced cancer. All such areas should be checked by a doctor.

Nipple Discharge

Nipple discharges, for the most part, are not associated with breast cancer, but they should be brought to the attention of your physician so that he can determine if treatment is necessary. A milky discharge from both breasts, apparent only after slight squeezing of the nipples, is associated with pregnancy and delivery and may persist for months or even years in some women after delivery. This is almost always a benign condition. Milky discharge from both breasts may also be due to medications, such as phenothiazine tranquilizers (Compazine, Stelazine, Thorazine), tricyclic antidepressants, oral contraceptives, and hypertension medications like rauwolfia compounds and methyldopa. It may also be part of some endocrine disorders, especially those associated with the absence of menses (amenorrhea-galactorrhea syndrome). Multicolored or yellow-green discharges that tend to be sticky are also most often caused by benign disease, usually an inflammation within the duct system of the breast.

Watery, pink, clear yellow, or bloody discharges are more rare, but they are the ones to be alert for. These are especially significant when they occur only in one breast and should be the basis for an immediate visit to your doctor. Your doctor can easily check while you are in his office for the presence of blood cells in the discharge. Even if there is blood, the cause is most likely to be a benign papilloma (overgrowth of the lining cells in the ducts). Sometimes, however, papillary carcinomas can be present. As with all other breast findings, the likelihood of cancer is increased with increasing age. No matter what your age is, however, a watery, clear yellow, or pink or bloody discharge of the breast should be thoroughly investigated.

The Postmenopausal Breast

In the postmenopausal breast, fibrous and cystic lumps tend to subside; a new lump that is found is more likely to be a cancer. Some women have the mistaken impression that after they are menopausal, they no longer need a yearly examination. Nothing could be further from the truth. The incidence of cancer increases with age, so the older you are, the more diligent you should be about your physical examinations.

Breast cancers tend not to be painful (as cysts often are because of the rapid increase of fluid pressure which causes stretching of the capsule, although there are exceptions to this rule). The cancer mass resists being moved when pushed with your fingers, and it is probably harder than other surrounding lumps in the breast. Breast cancers, for the most part, are hard because they are formed of tough, dense scar tissue. They might be thought of as scars in which the cancer cells are growing. (Most of the scar or fibrous tissue is the result of a defensive reaction of the body to the presence of the cancer.) These tumors are solid through and through. They are so solid that when they are removed and examined, the pathologist can not only cut them out neatly, but he can cut out a block shape with sharp corners. This type of common cancer is called scirrhous cancer.

Benign tumors do, however, occur in postmenopausal women. Many of them simulate cancers in the way they feel and by other breast changes that they cause. If you are postmenopausal and you find a lump, you will be a much more likely candidate for biopsy than a younger woman would be, simply because the risks of watching and waiting are too great. But there are women who have all the stigmata of breast cancer—including nipple discharge; nipple retraction; a stony, hard mass which may adhere to the skin— yet have a benign disease (for example, mammary-duct ectasia). Only a biopsy can determine which is which; survival depends on early detection in older women as much as in younger women.

In the postmenopausal breast, there also are soft tumors that are benign. These are fatty tumors called lipomas. Lipomas also occur in other parts of the body; in the breast, they are soft and completely nonsymptomatic. Let your doctor decide after examination and mammography (if indicated) whether biopsy is called for.

One more topic should be covered before leaving the discussion of breast disease in older women, and that is Paget's disease. It is a somewhat unusual form of cancer, because it produces early symptoms. These symptoms *first* involve the nipple. Patients complain of burning, itching, and discharge from the nipple and note that the nipple appears irritated, red, and wet. It seems like chronic eczema, for the nipple area weeps with a clear or slightly colored discharge and may have a scab or crust, especially if bacteria begin to infect the area. Many women believe that they have dermatitis, a skin problem, that simply will not clear up. Often they do not notice that the nipple is slowly being destroyed. If, however, the surrounding skin and other parts of your body are affected, you probably do have a dermatitis and not cancer. Paget's disease usually affects one breast, while dermatitis tends to affect both breasts at once; but you must consult your physician to have a proper evaluation. Paget's disease is special because it gives many early signals and can be cured. Many women, however, wait and apply salves for months, unaware that a cancer is growing. Sadly, this tumor, for all its warning signs, is usually brought to the attention of a surgeon only after long delays, usually for more than a year.

DEVELOPMENTS IN EARLY DETECTION

Among all these lumps and bumps, just about the smallest mass that can be discovered by breast self-examination is a cancerous tumor of 1 cubic centimeter ($\frac{1}{30}$ oz). A tumor of that small size already contains about one billion cancer cells. When an abnormal cancer cell divides, it produces two daughter cells which are also defective. Continuing cell division produces a growing malignancy that continues to multiply.

The estimated doubling time of mammary cancer—that is, the time in which the tumor doubles in size—varies from eighty-five days to fifteen months. Assuming that the doubling time remains constant at, for instance, a hundred days, it could take about eight years—or thirty doublings—for the growth to reach the size you can feel with your fingertips (1 cm^3). But it will then take only another hundred days to reach twice that size. This rapid logarithmic growth pattern makes early detection and immediate management of the cancer in its primary stages crucially important.

For this reason, researchers have been developing and refining new screening techniques that can find tiny tumors even before you can feel them with your fingers—before they have had a chance to spread. These new detection techniques can theoretically raise the survival rate to 95 percent. And that is good news indeed!

The first and the most controversial is mammography,

a special technique of taking breast X-rays that reveal the inner structure of the breast and its tumors, cysts, or distortions, if any. In 1976, the media reported that mammography increased the risk of breast cancer due to the effect of the X-rays on the breast. The scare headlines were a two-edged sword. On the positive side, doctors who had been indiscriminately prescribing these X-rays for women of all ages stopped doing so. On the negative side, the pendulum swung too far and nearly reversed all the progress that had been made in the field of early breast cancer detection. Patients were scared, and doctors became overcautious. No one had a good understanding of the risks as opposed to the benefits that patients would derive from mammography. Consequently, today many women who are at high risk and who need mammography are too frightened to use the procedure. This is unfortunate, because for high-risk women, the real benefits far outweigh the theoretical risks.

The media reports were based on the following research data: (1) women who had received multiple lung X-rays (fluoroscopy) during the treatment of tuberculosis were known to have increased rates of cancer; (2) women exposed to radiation when the atomic bomb was dropped in Japan had increased rates of cancer; and (3) women who underwent X-ray therapy to their breasts for breast inflammation after childbirth also showed increased incidence of breast cancer.

While there is no way of determining the precise risk of inducing breast cancer by mammography, it is possible to estimate that risk. The most commonly accepted estimate is that if one million women were to receive a 1-rad dose of radiation to their breasts—the radiation dose of most of the mammography machines now in use—six additional cases of breast cancer would occur per year. Since any woman already has a 7 percent chance of getting breast cancer (one woman out of fourteen), a single mammogram raises the risk by 0.07 percent to a 7.07 percent chance. If a woman has one mammogram a year for fifteen years, the risk factor will increase to 8 percent.

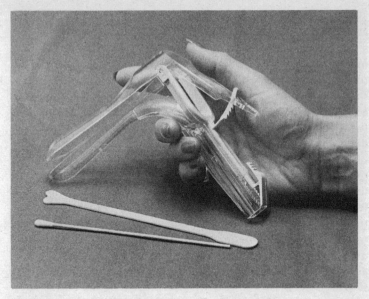

1. Speculum, cotton swab, and an Ayres spatula (wooden spatula) used for taking Pap smears.

2. Contraceptive foam: the filled applicator, ready for insertion.

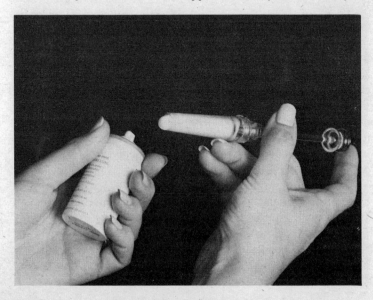

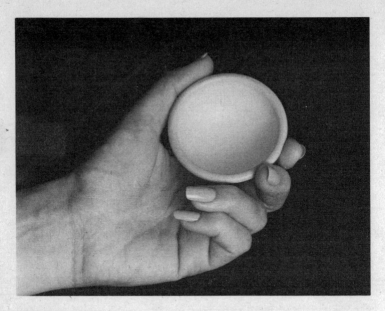

3a. Diaphragm.

3b. Applying contraceptive cream to diaphragm.

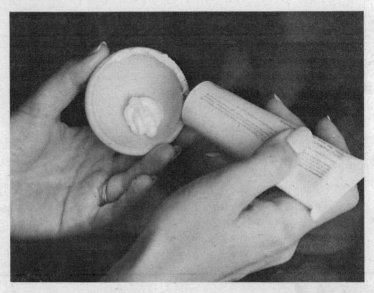

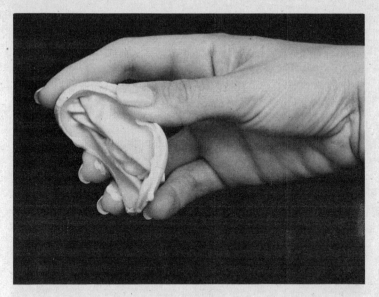

3c. Bending diaphragm to insert by hand.

3d. Using a diaphragm inserter. Some women find it easier, some more aesthetically pleasing.

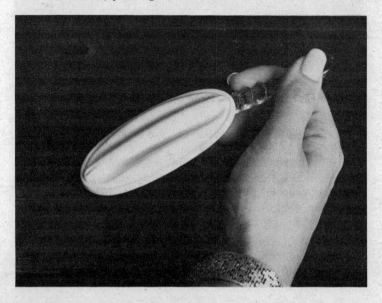

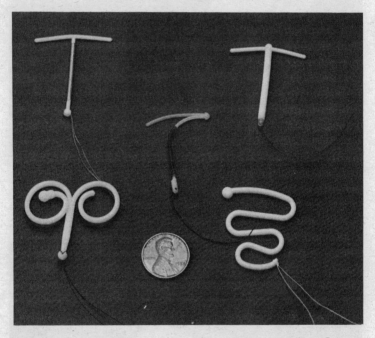

4. IUDs currently available in the United States: *Top left:* Tatum-T. Note copper wire wound about stem of T. *Top right:* Progestasert. Hollow stem contains progesterone. *Center:* Copper-7. Note copper wire wound about stem of 7. Wire appears dark, as copper has come off during three years' use of this device, just removed from a patient. *Bottom left:* Double spiral, inert device. *Bottom right:* Lippes Loop, inert device.

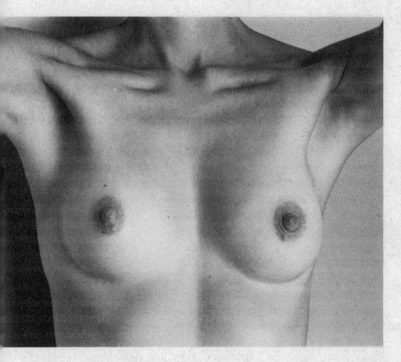

5. One of the most important things in breast self-examination is to flex your muscles and observe your breasts. Place your arms over your head and push your hands firmly together. This changes the contour of your breasts and may help you spot areas or changes that might otherwise have been missed.

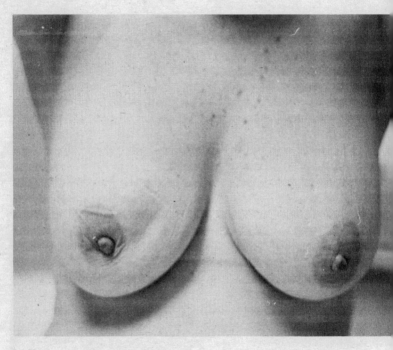

6. Compare right and left breasts. Note that right nipple is pulled inward and that there is an indentation in the skin produced by an underlying tumor.

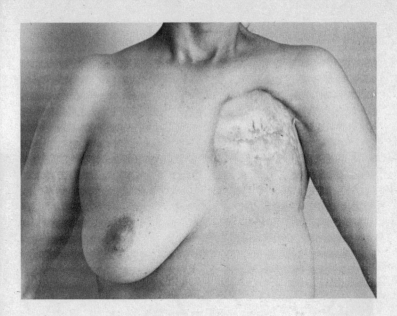

7a. Radical mastectomy (six years previously).

7b. Modified radical mastectomy.

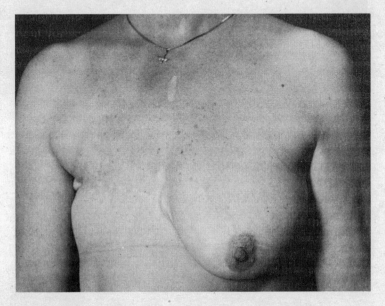

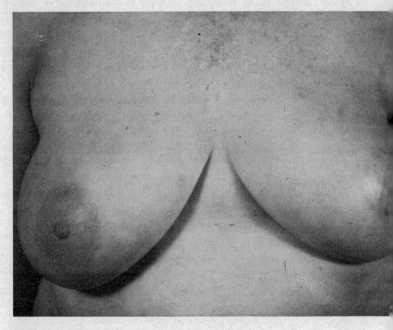

8. Post lumpectomy—left breast. Not all breasts may look this good, especially if the tumor is large, or if the breast is quite small.

However, even this risk factor can be decreased. The federal government is encouraging diagnostic centers and hospitals to update their facilities with newer machines which use only 0.2 to 0.3 rads per breast. The National Cancer Institute has established six regional Centers for Radiological Physics, which serve federally funded institutions. For nonfederally funded hospitals, the Bureau of Radiological Health of the FDA has developed a state-based Mammography Quality Assurance Program to minimize patient exposure and improve the image quality of X-rays. This program is known as Breast Exposure: Nationwide Trends (BENT). Unfortunately the program has no enforcement arm, but it has prevailed upon most doctors with high-dosage machines to stop taking X-rays or get new machines.

If you decide that you should have mammography, ask the radiologist about the radiation dosage of his machine. While the radiation dose you receive cannot be exactly determined beforehand, since it depends somewhat on the size and density of your breasts, you should at least be able to find out whether you will be exposed to an older machine using more than 1 rad per breast, or to one of the newer ones. If the radiologist is not available to tell you the dosages, don't hesitate to make further inquiries or to look elsewhere. In some localities, however, you may not have much of a choice.

General guidelines proposed by the American College of Radiology Committee on Mammography, and updated by the American Cancer Society, suggest mammography:

1. At any age, when your doctor's findings indicate a significant suspicion of cancer.
2. For women under the age of 35, only when there are specific, strong clinical indications; and for women 35–39 years of age, only when there is a personal history of breast cancer or if you desire a baseline mammography.
3. For women 40–49, if there is a personal history of breast cancer in first-degree relatives—that is, mother or sister—or if you desire a baseline mammography.

4. For women 50 and over, annual or biannual preventative screening is statistically justifiable.

Most radiologists feel that women should have a baseline mammographic study at age 50. Others opt for doing the study when the woman is in her 40s, or between 35 and 40, but all agree that a baseline study should be done. Having a "normal" picture of your breast anatomy can be extremely helpful in interpreting subtle changes that might occur in the future. In addition, although the purpose of baseline studies is to give a picture of normal breasts, these studies help to detect a small but significant number of early cancers. There also is some evidence that the radiologic appearance of breast patterns can be used as an indicator of higher or lower cancer-risk categories, although this evidence is now being hotly debated by two well-known and respected radiologists.

While the risks of mammography should not be minimized, there is considerable evidence that mammography can detect a tumor as long as two years before it is possible to find it by palpation, or manual examination. That's an important edge that has a direct relationship to survival. Recent improvements in mammography have sharpened images and made the films more detailed, thereby increasing further the chances of finding small tumors.

Unfortunately, mammograms are not infallible. Approximately 10 to 15 percent of breast cancers do not show up on the film. Mammograms are especially difficult to read on younger women, whose dense, glandular tissue sometimes masks tumors. If you have a mass that is palpable, and yet your mammogram is negative, your doctor should be guided by his clinical judgment and order a biopsy if he is at all suspicious. Every physician has been misled at one time or another by placing too much reliance on X-ray reports.

For the younger woman with a suspicious mass, a newer technique, *xerography,* may be more reliable. Xerography uses a different X-ray process that results in a positive blue-on-white photographic print rather than a negative shadowgram, as in mammography. Thus xerography better defines dense breasts, but it uses slightly more radiation than the newer mammography techniques.

Breast Cancer Risk Factors and Mammography

If you are between the ages of 35 and 49, here are the risk factors that can help you make up your mind whether to have a mammogram. The more risk factors you have, the greater the chance of breast cancer. (Any suspicious mass, of course, should be biopsied—*no matter what your mammogram shows.*)

a previous breast cancer
a mother who developed breast cancer in both breasts when
    she was still premenopausal
a mother with breast cancer
a sister with breast cancer
previous multiple chest fluoroscopies (for tuberculosis, etc.)
several members of your family afflicted with cancer (ovarian,
    endometrial, stomach, colon, etc.)
other previous cancers (uterine or ovarian)

Less important factors:

history of cystic breast disease
very large breasts (simply because it is difficult to find a
    lump in a full breast, especially a lump that might be
    deep within the breast)
childlessness, or birth of your first child when you were
    30 years old or older
menstruation begun at or before age 11
overweight (especially from a high fat diet)

Most important factors at any age:

a noticeable change in your breast, whether or not a mass is palpable. For example: recent onset of nipple retraction; thickening or skin changes in a portion of the breast; nipple discharge that is clear or bloody; a firm lymph node in the armpit. These are indications of possible cancer; you should consult a doctor immediately.

You can determine the risk factors that apply to yourself. Although no individual prediction can be made, the more factors that are present, the greater your chances for one day having breast cancer. If you are in a high-risk category, you must examine yourself regularly and see your doctor twice a year.

When mammography has identified a lesion but cannot delineate whether the lesion is benign or malignant, many surgeons do and should do a biopsy. Others, however, may try one of the newer X-ray techniques that have been developed to supplement mammography and xerography and lead to more specific conclusions.

One of the newer techniques, *scintigraphy,* makes use of a radioactive material (technetium 99), which is injected into a vein in your arm. The material is picked up and concentrated in the breast tissue. Because malignant tumors usually grow more rapidly than benign tumors and the surrounding tissue, they will absorb more of the radioactive material and show up as hot spots on the machine display. Scintigraphy is used mainly to supplement and provide further definition of a mass picked up on a mammogram rather than to take the place of mammography.

Another X-ray technique that will probably be widely available soon is the Computed Tomography (CT) *breast scan.* This scan technique involves the injection of an iodine solution. Normal breast tissue absorbs only small amounts, but cancerous tissue absorbs large amounts and shows up vividly on the exposed film. One of the advantages of the technique is that the CT scan can often differentiate between fibrocystic disease and cancer. It can also distinguish between normal postoperative (breast biopsy or lumpectomy) changes that occur in the breast and residual cancer. Because this test involves the intake of a foreign substance (iodine) into the bloodstream, it is not appropriate for use as a mass screening tool because severe allergic reactions are possible. Therefore, it is limited to use in high-risk patients or patients who have multiple lesions where one or more could be malignant.[7]

Nonradiation Methods of Detection

In addition to the techniques that use X-rays or radiation, other methods of early detection are available that do not involve radiation. One is *thermography,* a process that takes a photograph of the heat patterns on the surface of the breast. Abnormalities of the breast show up as hot spots on the photograph. Thermography may be appropriate for screening younger women, who should not be exposed to radiation. Unfortunately it is unreliable, since the thermogram may be interpreted differently by different doctors, or even by the same doctor on different days. Recently computers have been used to interpret the results, and they may completely take over the task of interpretation from people in the near future. Computers always interpret the same way, with or without their morning coffee.

Given the current state of the art, thermography is not accurate enough to be a definitive diagnostic test and should never be used as such. The American Cancer Society recommends its use for women between the ages of 35 and 50 who are not in the high-risk group as part of a complete annual physical examination. If a hot spot shows up on the thermogram, a mammogram can be done to more accurately determine if the hot spot is a tumor. In this way, only those women who really should be checked out need be exposed to radiation. However, because of the inaccuracy of thermography, it is no longer used as a routine procedure in Breast Cancer Detection Demonstration Projects.

Another technique currently under investigation—*ultrasound*—involves the use of high-frequency sound waves rather than X-rays. Sonography, as this technique is called, is another painless noninvasive method of detecting breast abnormalities.

The patient lies face down on a specially constructed bed, with her breasts hanging through an opening and completely immersed in a tank of water. High-frequency sound waves are projected into the breast, and the pattern of echoes they produce is converted by a computer into an image that shows the different densities of the interior of the breast. Various studies are now being conducted to determine the safety and accuracy of ultrasound. The procedure is advancing rapidly as new refinements in equipment are developed. In the fall of 1979, doctors at the Mount Sinai Medical Center in Miami Beach reported that a new waterbath ultrasound technique designed expressly for breast imagery proved to be as effective as mammography in detecting cancer of the breast. The Miami researchers, as well as a group at Thomas Jefferson University, feel that ultrasound will soon become the preferred procedure in screening for breast cancer. It promises to show excellent detail and be free of the intrinsic dangers of radiation associated with mammography.

This news certainly is encouraging, but it will take time for other ultrasonographers to be as well trained in interpreting the images as are the doctors who did the pilot study. It will also take time to manufacture and distribute the very sophisticated ultrasound equipment.

In the meantime, the type of screening exam that you get will depend mostly on what is available in your area. And what is available depends in large measure on the technique the radiologist was trained in and is most comfortable with, and on the equipment he has to work with. In spite of all the marvelous technology that is being developed, the fact of the matter is that we do not, as yet, have a definitive screening test for positively identifying breast cancer 100 percent of the time.

However, some very encouraging work is now being done in research laboratories, the most promising of which is in the field of blood analysis. Researchers are working on the theory that a specific substance in the blood (known as antigen or tumor marker) indicates the presence of breast cancer. They are attempting to develop a blood test that will show when the antigen is present, which would indicate that a tumor was developing in the breast. If they are successful, breast-cancer screening will be a simple matter of sending blood specimens to the laboratory for analysis. This blood test will have the potential of earlier and more accurate detection than any means of screening now available. It will detect abnormal cancer cells before a visible or palpable mass is present, when the body may be able to wipe out the intruders with its own powerful defenses and the help of low-dosage drugs. When such a test is developed, we will have taken a giant step forward in the battle against breast cancer.

Of all these recent technological developments directed at early detection of breast cancer, some are available now and some will come in the near future. But they will be ineffective for many women, because advances are useless if women will not have semiannual or annual exams that include a breast check and examine their own breasts on a monthly basis. At this point, no one can say which particular detection procedure is the most reliable, but we do know that the sooner a cancerous lump is found, the better are your chances both for survival and for nondisfiguring surgery. So the best advice I can give you for early detection of breast cancer is:

1. Learn and practice breast self-examination.
2. Have an annual checkup performed by a physician who takes the time to do a thorough breast examination. If you are over 40, you should have a physical examination twice a year and a baseline mammogram.
3. If you are 50 or older, have an annual or biannual mammogram and a semiannual checkup.
4. If you are in a high-risk group, have a baseline mammogram sometime between the ages of 35 and 49 and a semiannual checkup.

If you have cystic breasts, cut down on tea, chocolate, brown-colored sodas and caffeinated coffee. All of these contain methylxanthines (which includes caffeine) that probably contribute to breast cysts by stimulating the breast cells to overproduce tissue and cyst fluid. Because cysts make breasts tender and difficult to palpate, and often result in increased biopsies, you may be interested in a recent study conducted by Dr. Minton et al.[8]

Forty-seven women with fibrocystic breast disease were instructed to stop their intake of coffee, tea, brown sodas and chocolate. These women previously drank an average of four cups of coffee per day. Of the group, twenty totally stopped. Of these, thirteen experienced the complete disappearance of all of their palpable lumps within one to six months. Only one of the twenty-seven women who continued to drink coffee experienced resolution of her breast lumps.

Long-term follow-up of these patients showed that the women who restricted their consumption of drinks containing methylxanthines continued to have normal breasts for as long as they abstained, but the disease rapidly returned when they resumed their old coffee-drinking habits. Dr. Minton mentioned one other factor. Three of the seven patients who restricted their coffee intake, but "whose disease did not resolve have had significant resolution since they stopped smoking. Complete resolution of disease required a year or more in women 45 years and older."

Though the numbers in this study are small, this observation, if substantiated by future better controlled studies, may have wide repercussions for the coffee-drinking United States. Meanwhile, I have been impressed enough by this first bit of evidence to recommend that my patients with cystic breasts either stop their coffee, tea, cola and chocolate habits, or at least cut down.

It is important to remember that even though it seems that caffeine and other methylxanthines contribute to the formation of breast cysts, no studies have ever proved that caffeine contributes to the development of breast cancer.

DIAGNOSIS AND TREATMENT

When the results of all the diagnostic tests indicate the presence of cancer, the physician must use these findings and the clinical examination to determine the stage or spread of the disease. Therefore, lymph nodes are removed during surgery primarily to see if the cancer cells have spread and invaded that far—this helps to "stage" the cancer and determines the most appropriate treatment and general prognosis.

The clinical stages, in abbreviated form, are:

Stage I: breast cancer in the earliest stage is confined to the breast, with no apparent spread to the armpit lymph glands.

Stage II: lymph nodes in the armpit are enlarged and firm and may contain cancerous cells that have spread from the breast.

Stage III: large tumors, or tumors that have spread to the armpit, above the clavicle, or become fixed to the underlying chest muscle are present; but cancer apparently has not spread to other distant parts of the body.

Stage IV: distant metastases are present. That is, the tumor has spread to the bone, liver, or other distant parts of the body.

Another dimension may be added to clinical staging by the increasing evidence that prostaglandins are involved in breast cancer. Some years ago, Dr. Alan Bennett discovered that patients with the highest amounts of prostaglandin in a tumor had the worst life expectancies.[9] It is possible, then, that prostaglandin levels may be used to refine our estimates of how long the patient will live and how soon she should receive additional therapy. This refinement could be very helpful, for merely feeling and looking—the mainstays of the present clinical staging process—are still fairly primitive ways of predicting prognosis.

There may be other criteria for prognosis, such as the pathologist's microscopic interpretation, which may confirm whether or not the cancer appears to be aggressive, or if it has invaded the lymphatics or the blood vessels. These observations are often more important than the size of the original tumor or its local spread, and may help to explain why some women with small tumors do poorly, while other women with larger tumors outlive them by many years. Blood-vessel invasion should alert us to the fact that early spread of the tumor may occur.

In the early stages of the disease, surgical procedures are performed in the hope of potential cure; but Stage III and IV patients, who have severe involvement or who are likely to have distant metastases, are not thought of as good candidates for cure by surgery. For carefully selected Stage III and IV patients, simple palliative surgery may be performed to reduce the tumor burden, relieve local distressing symptoms, and make the patient more comfortable in the advanced stages of the disease. Only in Stages I and II of the disease are surgical procedures considered able to effect a cure. Luckily, half the breast cancers are now being detected in Stage I (before there is any spread to the nodes), and 35 percent are detected in Stage II.

At these early stages, there are several different surgical options, and surgeons wrangle continuously among themselves about which procedure is best. Every surgeon would agree that once a cancer has spread to an area of the body other than the breast, surgery cannot possibly "cure" the patient. Yet they disagree about how much surgery should be performed initially for Stage I and II cancers. Each is convinced, based on his own personal experience and what he has been taught, that he is right and the others are wrong. What this difference of opinion among surgeons really means is that none of them knows the answer. If any of the procedures provided a 100 percent cure rate, obviously all surgeons would immediately adopt that procedure. But there is no one procedure that stands so obviously above the others.

Ideally, surgery should not be the treatment of choice for any disease. The surgical removal of a breast or any other organ that has been invaded by cancer is an admission that doctors don't understand cancer, what causes it, how to prevent it, or how to control it in a more sophisticated, specific way. But at the present time, except for primary radiation (discussed in detail on pages 176–79), there is no proven alternative to surgery for women with diagnosed Stage I or II breast cancer. For many women, then, the question becomes not whether to have surgery, but how much surgery to have.

Certainly the time has come to discard the 80-year-old surgical technique of radical mastectomy called the Halsted procedure. In his day, at the turn of the century, Halsted was one of the best things that happened to women. Then the practice of surgery was just beginning to bloom because of the discovery of anesthesia, which made possible procedures far more prolonged than the swiftest of amputations. Little was known about the way cancer grew and spread or of the importance of doing surgery early in the disease process. In those days, breast cancer was thought of as a venereal disease, and most patients suffered in silence as if they were doing penance for their sins. Women were reluctant to come forward until their lesions made life unbearable. Many women who came to Halsted had huge lesions that often had spread to their lymph nodes, but his meticulous surgical skill saved the lives of some fortunate women who still had early disease and prolonged the lives of many others.

Halsted's operation became justly famous. Because Halsted believed that every vestige of the cancer must be removed to prevent its spread, his procedure involved removing the entire breast, the underlying chest muscles, and the under-arm lymph nodes all in one piece. He left the patient with a thin, bony chest wall by making sure that he took out all remnants of muscle and fat. In time, Halsted extended his surgery so that he also removed the lymph nodes at the base of the neck. When he noted that this extended procedure did not increase the life expectancy of the patient, he abandoned it.

From an esthetic point of view, radical mastectomy was—and still is—a disaster. It leaves the chest wall looking skeletonlike, with the hollowness extending all the way to the collarbone on the affected side. Small wonder these women complain about chest pain from the cold on a winter day. Without its usual muscle and fat protection, the rib cage and the inside of the body are mercilessly exposed to temperature variations. Patients suffer shoulder stiffness and weakness of the affected arm because of the large amount of muscle removed. They also experience swelling of the involved arm because of poor fluid drainage (due to removal of most of the armpit nodes), and they become extremely susceptible to infection from the slightest nick or scratch to the affected extremity. In the 1890s, however, it was Halsted or certain death.

In the United States, the merits of the Halsted radical mastectomy remained undisputed; but in 1948, two British surgeons who believed that leaving the chest muscles intact would not affect the spread of the disease began using a lesser surgical technique, called the modified radical. This involved removing the entire breast and some fat and most of the axillary nodes, but left the chest muscle intact. (It appears that their assumption that cancer does not spread through the chest muscles is correct. If the chest muscles become involved, the cancer is far advanced, and surgery is not the appropriate treatment.) In the modified radical procedure, the incision itself is also less disfiguring because it is horizontal and does not extend upward toward the collarbone. Furthermore, the chest is left well padded with muscle (like a man's chest), so that women can wear clothes with cut-out necklines. Because the muscles are preserved, the arms have good strength. Women have fewer problems with swelling because fewer nodes are removed, causing less damage to the arm's fluid-drainage system. Moreover, these women are ideal candidates for plastic reconstruction at a future date, if they so desire.

Also in 1948, Dr. Robert McWhirter reported that the survival rates for patients treated by simple mastectomy, in which just the breast is removed and the axillary nodes and muscle are left intact, followed by radiation, were essentially the same as those for patients treated with the Halsted radical mastectomy plus radiation.

Dr. McWhirter's findings were confirmed by a British study begun in 1967 and by a clinical trial begun in 1971 by the National Surgical Adjuvant Breast Project (NSABP). These studies showed no advantage in recurrence rates or survival rates for patients who had undergone the Halsted radical mastectomy as compared to patients who had undergone simple mastectomy and radiation.

McWhirter's patients did not suffer from swelling of their arms because the lymphatic drainage from the arm is not disturbed. Furthermore, the possibility of easy infection of the arm was not an ever-present danger after his procedure.

McWhirter did not biopsy the nodes to determine if they were affected, because he believed that even the most radical surgery failed to eliminate all cancer in the operative area. He concluded that radiation therapy would destroy the cancerous cells that remained in the operative area, as well as those in the nodes.[10]

In the late 1950s, some daring surgeons performed partial mastectomies during which the tumor and two to three centimeters of the surrounding tissue were removed, leaving the remainder of the breast intact. This was usually followed by radiation therapy to kill any cancer cells that remained in the breast. Despite the anguished cries of their more conventional colleagues that these surgeons were sentencing their patients to sure death, studies showed that the survival rates from partial mastectomy—or "lumpectomy"—are about the same as for total mastectomy.

Lumpectomy is just that—removal of the tumor lump and only a small amount of surrounding tissue. The amount removed depends upon the surgeon. Some surgeons take a minimal area around the tumor, while others claiming to do a lumpectomy are actually taking a fair portion of the breast or even performing a quadrantectomy, which removes the quarter of the breast containing the tumor. The physician may also remove lymph nodes from the axilla (armpit) for analysis and prognosis. Then radiation—given in slow doses over a five- to nine-week period—may be used to "sterilize" the remaining breast tissue, in case small amounts of tumor are still present. Studies currently being done in Boston and on Long Island show excellent survival rates for patients with early breast disease and minimal surgery. The success in treating Stage I and II cancers by simple tumor removal and radiation have made doctors more aware that lesser surgery may be as beneficial as the old-fashioned mutilating surgery.

For many years, European medical textbooks regarded the Halsted radical mastectomy as an operation to be aware of *only* because of its historical significance. Yet eighty years after its development, the Halsted radical is still used in this country in *one-quarter* of all breast surgery. Actually, Halsted probably would turn over in his grave if he knew that his name was attached to the present-day radical mastectomy. Halsted spent nearly five hours on each case, meticulously looking, feeling, and dissecting. No surgeon today does a true Halsted, because he can't afford the time or the anesthesia risk to do such an extended, unnecessarily time-consuming procedure.

I would never consent to a radical mastectomy for myself. I have given the matter a good deal of thought, because as I advise others, I always consider what I would do if I were in the same situation. I have had my share of patients who have undergone surgery. I have listened to surgeons who painstakingly explain that the radical is the only proven method and, therefore, the one which is the standard for all comparisons. I think that the radical mastectomy has had too long a trial in this country. I and everyone else know that the statistics for the radical operation are unsatisfactory.

The surgeons have picked a poor yardstick by which to measure other procedures. I would choose not to be sacrificed as yet another case to prove that the statistics with the Halsted are unacceptable. Because lesser surgery achieves a similar survival rate, I would choose the least amount of surgery. To me, that means a lumpectomy and probably postoperative radiation.

As a woman, I can cope with that. As a physician, I feel it would be an appropriate and logical choice.

Whatever surgical procedure you choose, I suggest some presurgical guidelines. First of all, I recommend that my patients consent only to a diagnostic biopsy and deny written permission for the combined biopsy/mastectomy that is so popular with so many surgeons. During that combined procedure, the surgeon sends the biopsy specimen to the pathologist, who quick-freezes it, takes a slice, and reads it—all while the patient is on the operating table. If the pathologist finds cancer, the surgeon completes the mastectomy. If not, no further surgery is performed.

I have always felt that this combined procedure, while it is very convenient for the surgeon, leaves room for irreversible error and needlessly subjects patients—most of whom will prove *not* to have cancer—to anxiety and fear. In my 1976 "Women in Industry" speech, I said so:

> Eight out of ten of these women do not have cancer, yet we subject them to all of the emotional trauma. They should be able to have their biopsies without spending the night crying into their pillows for fear of mutilation. There is no terror of a "little biopsy," which may even be done on an outpatient basis, possibly with no anesthesia other than the dental-type local Novocain. Most women can face up to that. Most women would welcome such a biopsy to rid their mind of the terrible fear that lurks there.
>
> My patients initially give consent for biopsy of the suspicious area only. They know they will awaken from surgery with their breast intact. If the lesion is benign, they are home free. They

have not been unnecessarily put through the terrible fear of losing their breast. Should the biopsy prove to be malignant, the patient has time to put her thoughts together, talk over her future surgery, prepare her own personal defenses, and consider possible alternatives. She retains control of her body and does not face the shock and anger of having been assured that "all will be well," only to wake up to the fact that not only does she have cancer, but she has been mutilated as well.[11]

In 1979, the panel of cancer specialists convened by the National Cancer Institute endorsed this two-step procedure.

In my judgment, a one-step biopsy-and-surgery procedure might be used only when the contemplated curative surgery is a lumpectomy. If the biopsy shows a lump to be malignant, it might as well be totally removed right away; and waking up without a lump is much different from waking up without a breast. But if you would rather not even think about the possible surgical variations until the biopsy is over, insist on a two-step procedure.

The value of biopsy under local anesthesia is becoming increasingly apparent to many surgeons. In fact, surgeons are beginning to do needle biopsies and to remove some nodules in their offices. As there are no bones to saw through and no muscle to cut through, a tiny scalpel and a one-to two-inch incision enable the surgeon to reach the lump and remove it. Depending on the size of the incision and how close together he places the sutures, three to six stitches are all that it usually takes to repair the incision, and you go home with little more than a Band-Aid. Generally, the surgeon will send the biopsy to the same pathologist who would read the specimen if it had been removed in the hospital operating room, and the pathology report is usually back in forty-eight hours. Somehow having a biopsy done in the doctor's office or even in an emergency room is less scary than being admitted to a hospital.

If for some reason you do decide to give consent for a combined biopsy/mastectomy, you should have certain tests done and the results entered in your hospital record before you go into the operating room. Such tests can rule out the distant spread of the disease before surgery is performed. (If the disease has metastasized, surgery should be minimal and only done for biopsy or palliative purposes.) To proceed with curative surgery, you must have the following test results:

1. *Normal results in blood tests.* Abnormal blood-test results could reflect metastases, especially in the liver or bone. Some of the important blood tests are a CBC (Complete Blood Count) and bone and liver tests (alkaline phosphotase, SGOT, SGPT, bilirubin); all are included in the comprehensive SMA-12 blood test.
2. *Normal results in urinalysis.*
3. *Normal chest X-ray.* This rules out metastases to the lungs.
4. *Normal bone scan.* This rules out distant metastases to bone.
5. *Normal results in gynecological examination.* This insures that there is no spread of the breast cancer to the ovaries.
6. *Normal liver scan.* This rules out spread to the liver.

Whether a liver scan is essential prior to surgery is debatable. Since breast tumors usually spread to bone first and later to the liver, many surgeons feel that if the bone scan is normal, the liver scan is unnecessary. This is especially likely to be true when blood tests show that the liver function is normal. I am somewhat less cost conscious, however, and always order a liver scan on my patients who are scheduled for mastectomy. This initial study serves as a baseline for the comparison of future scans. Once or twice, I was chagrined to find that this baseline liver scan was not normal and that the tumor had already spread. Therefore, it was too late to do curative surgery.

Another patient had an initially confusing liver scan which did not appear to be caused by a metastatic disease. After careful questioning, I discovered that the patient had had a transfusion years ago, and concluded that she most likely had contracted a case of undetected hepatitis. If I had not obtained that initial scan, but had done a scan only years later when she complained of symptoms, the peculiar pattern might have been misinterpreted, and the patient could have received unnecessary treatment.

ESTROGEN RECEPTORS

If you have to undergo surgery for breast cancer, it is vital that arrangements be made before your surgery for an estrogen-receptor test. Your surgeon, the laboratory, and the pathologist must understand and agree to the test so that it can become part of your surgical procedure. The knowledge gained from the test will do little to influence your immediate therapy, but it will be extremely important if your tumor should spread years later to another part of your body. If your breast tumor contains estrogen receptors, new tumors that develop elsewhere in the body will probably also have these same qualities. If further therapy is necessary, then hormonal manipulation rather than chemotherapy should be used. The test can assure that you will receive the most effective treatment and prevent you from receiving therapy that will most likely not work. If you have positive estrogen-receptor sites, it also implies that your overall prognosis is better than if your receptor sites are estrogen-negative.

RADIATION THERAPY

It is apparent that while medical science has not been very effective in improving overall breast-cancer survival rates, it has succeeded in reducing the disfigurement involved in treatment while at the same time not diminishing the survival rate. This has been accomplished by combining radiation with surgery or by using radiation alone after biopsy to avoid the more radical mutilating surgery.

Studies are being conducted in which breast cancer after biopsy is being treated by radiation alone. The *Breast Cancer*

Digest of the United States Department of Health, Education and Welfare reports that

> Radiation therapy is an effective form of treatment for many types of cancer. . . . Many physicians now believe radiation is as effective as mastectomy in treating breast cancer when used alone or combined with local excision.

The *Journal of Reproductive Medicine* reports that surgery for breast cancer has "neither significantly improved the curability of the disease nor decreased its posttreatment morbidity." On the other hand,

> radical radiation therapy is a viable alternative to radical mastectomy in early breast cancer, and the radiation therapy in combination with surgery significantly improves both the quality and the duration of life in women with breast cancer.[12]

Early attempts at radiation treatment were less effective because the radiation dosages were too small, but eventually doctors learned that higher doses of radiation were necessary to kill the cancer cells by preventing them from dividing. These higher doses effectively eliminated most cancer recurrences near the site of the original tumor. Today there are several long-term studies underway comparing the survival rates of patients treated by surgery and patients treated by radiation; and while some experts agree that the studies have not yet gone on long enough, the results so far indicate that survival rates of the two groups are similar.

Radiation therapy can be given completely externally or by internal implants placed directly into the tumor area after the tumor itself has been removed for biopsy. Dr. Samuel Hellman of the Department of Radiation Therapy at Harvard Medical School cites studies that show that interstitial radiation implant therapy in combination with external radiation yields survival rates that are "quite comparable" to those of surgical procedures among patients with Stage I and II disease.

Reminding physicians that putting radioactive implants directly into a tumor is a fifty-year-old technique, he reported on a series of 176 patients who were treated by implants and with external radiation. "Five-year survival rates for this group of patients were 91 percent for those with Stage I breast cancer and 68 percent for those with Stage II cancer." He states, "I tell my patients that this is not an experimental procedure. We just know a lot less about it than we know about mastectomy."

In his current work, Hellman is combining high-energy X-ray, which he calls supervoltage radiation, with interstitial implants and says that so far, the results are again "quite comparable to those obtained with surgery alone." No major complications have appeared in 184 patients during a follow-up period of two to twelve years.

Women who undergo modern radiation therapy have cosmetically acceptable breasts after their treatment. As the tumor regresses, it is replaced by fibrous tissue, often leaving the breast somewhat smaller and firmer than it was before radiation. This is not always undesirable. One of my patients was so pleased with the shape and new firmness of her newly radiated breast that she kidded the radiotherapist about radiating her normal breast. (The radiotherapist has proudly told that story at least a hundred times.)

Unfortunately, many physicians and surgeons are not aware of many of the new developments in radiation treatment. The chief of surgery at a highly respected teaching medical center, with whom I discussed radiation, still thought that radiation shriveled the breast and completely ruined its appearance. If that chief of surgery had antiquated ideas, you can bet that other surgeons at smaller hospitals are also not up to date. And if they subject a patient to rapid radiation, the breast tissue may indeed become very fibrous and hard. Other complications of radiation include some skin discoloration, slight cough or chest achiness, and rare occurrences of rib fractures due to the effect of radiation on the bone structure.

Women who have undergone radiation therapy, just like

postmastectomy patients, must continue to see their doctors to be sure that there is no recurrence of the disease. This usually involves mammography or ultrasonography to assess both the postradiation breast and the unaffected breast. These tests can follow the shrinkage of the tumor and its replacement by the newly growing fibrous tissue. Any new disease should be picked up on routine follow-up mammography.

HOW TO GET WHAT YOU WANT

Women must have the final choice as to how much surgery—if any—they will have. You should keep in mind, however, that the choice of minimal surgery may be impractical if your breast contains more than one malignant area. If three definite lumps are palpable or one major lump is present in a breast with marked fibrocystic disease (that is, the breast is so lumpy that the surgeon can't tell which of many lumps is potentially bad), then total mastectomy (simple removal of only the breast, leaving muscle and lymph nodes) may be the least mutilating procedure that can be chosen. If the lesion is just under the nipple, or if the lump is very large and the breast is very small, a lumpectomy may leave the breast looking so damaged that, for cosmetic reasons, a simple mastectomy would be a better choice. But keep in mind that on the whole, breast surgery is neither complicated nor difficult for the surgeon, since he is working on a surface area with tissue that is soft and completely separated from any vital organs.

Make sure that the surgeon fully discusses with you all the available alternatives. This is easier said than done. Few surgeons will be enthusiastic about reviewing all the possible procedures for you. Should they do so, they will slant the presentation in favor of their favorite. Therefore, you should consider all the evidence and draw your own conclusions. Sometimes you may have to read between the lines or be aware of the omissions in his presentation. And it is quite likely that it will be difficult to find a surgeon willing to perform a lumpectomy. Since it is the newest procedure, many surgeons don't do it. They may fear that if a patient dies of cancer sometime after lumpectomy, they may be sued for not performing a more radical operation.

Your surgeon has neither the right nor the capacity to judge the psychological needs that form the basis of your final decision. A doctor performs a service for which he is paid—much like a plumber or an interior decorator. You are also paying him for his medical/surgical advice, but you know your own needs better than anyone else in the world. You must remember at this critical time that your doctor is *not* your father. Judgments are left to fathers; scientific fact is for doctors. In the final analysis, it is you who must select the procedure that you will be most comfortable with psychologically.

Your surgeon may insinuate that if you don't leave your fate in his hands, the outcome will be bad. This is the worst possible time in your life to feel so completely helpless; don't be pressured into making a decision that you may regret. You must make your own choice, for you will live with the consequences for the rest of your life. If, after examining all the possibilities, you decide that a lumpectomy is what you want, then that's what your surgeon should do. If he won't consider your choice, look for another surgeon and get another opinion.

Surgeons are not villains, but their training prepared them for blood and guts, to be cool and unflappable in all situations, and to make split-second decisions. Their field has overspecialized them and made them forget that beneath that diseased breast there is a real person with real fears and feelings. For the most part, surgeons do not like to be bothered with small talk. Furthermore, they usually feel that they know best and that their surgical preference is the best for all their patients. Consequently, as far as they are concerned, there really isn't anything to talk about.

The reason for this attitude may be that they are more comfortable doing one procedure than another. Perhaps the surgeon spent his residency being trained by another surgeon who favored radicals. The lesson stuck and became part of his repertoire. Just as a tennis player will not change rackets for fear of ruining his game, surgeons would rather perform a well-learned procedure than break in a new one. Furthermore, because he knows the procedure so well, he is convinced it is best for his patients. Sooner or later, patients too become convinced that what the surgeon recommends has got to be the best. But is it?

Medical literature is being enriched daily with more studies confirming that the difference in survival rates between the various treatments for breast cancer is negligible or even nonexistent at five years. In fact, it seems that most of the lesser methods have equal statistics at five years.

More "good news" is reported from Italy in a breast-tumor study involving 701 women, half of whom received the Halsted radical mastectomy, and the other half a lumpectomy and radiation. The total survival rates were 89.7 for the radical and 88.5 percent for the lumpectomy. The cancer-free survival rates were 83 percent for the Halsted group and 82.7 percent for the lumpectomy group. These five-year statistics are nearly identical and demonstrate that one procedure has no statistical advantage over the other.[13]

Five-year survival rates with excision biopsy and radiation or lumpectomy and radiation are as good as survival rates with the standard radical mastectomy. I believe that in patients with Stage I and II disease, radiation and lumpectomy have the same potential to wipe out disease in the breast as does modified radical or radical surgery. Will there be a great disparity between the survival figures at ten and twenty years? We don't know yet, but I personally am convinced from the growing data that the ten- and twenty-year survival rates will continue to be as good. On the other hand, if you cannot feel comfortable with the fact that a large amount of data does not yet exist, you should consider surgery that removes the entire breast.

We can read about statistics until we are tired of turning pages, but statistics will never tell us the quality of life or the quality of survival. For many a woman, the quality of life and the quality of survival will be best with an intact body. A radiation or lumpectomy patient can be assured that her five-year survival will be similar to that of a mastectomy patient. However, her ten-year survival might not be; it might be worse, it might be better. But another factor to consider is that in five years, there may be a revolution in breast-cancer therapy. Why not be optimistic and keep your breast until then?

Keep in mind that medical science is constantly advancing. For instance, for years, we amputated limbs of patients with bone tumors, but currently, these patients are often treated with chemotherapy plus wide resection of the bone. Not only do they keep their arms and legs, but with chemotherapy, they are better off than they ever were with amputation.

Surgery is a treatment method that is useful only until a better method of dealing with a disease is developed. Antibiotics have eliminated mastoid surgery, major tranquilizers have ended almost all brain psychosurgery, and antidiabetic drugs have put an end to some amputations for gangrene: drugs closely related to the prostaglandins are now in experimental use that have very positive results in increasing blood flow to blood-starved, nearly gangrenous legs. Doctors in Krakow, Poland, have accomplished some astonishing changes in such limbs and have prevented amputation.[14] Doses of antiprostaglandins have been used to cure heart defects in babies, thus sparing them major heart surgery.

I am convinced that a similar situation soon will occur in the case of breast cancer. Perhaps interferon will give us that breakthrough. Another few years may provide enough information to swing medical thinking away from surgery altogether.

In the meantime, surgeons are at least going to have to learn to talk to their patients. In fact, the state of Massachusetts has passed a law requiring surgeons to discuss with their patients all the options for treating breast cancer or be liable for malpractice. This means that they must go through an explanation of radiation therapy and lumpectomy as well as radical mastectomy. The law cannot dictate how they slant their descriptions, but at least Massachusetts women will know that choices exist. Perhaps that will help avoid the depression so many women have suffered after a mastectomy, depression that I believe to be masked anger against the surgeon for mutilating them. Depression is, after all, nothing more than anger that we cannot express turned against ourselves.

For their part, women are going to have to learn to talk to their doctors and to firmly assert their right to information and choice. But that may not be as easy as it sounds, for even as a doctor, I have trouble enough trying to make my male colleagues understand a female point of view. I remember when, several years ago, I was trying desperately to find a surgeon who would consent to do less than a radical on my patients. My discussions with most surgeons were short—"No." I still recall approaching one surgeon whom I felt might be more pliable. He stood in the hallway of the hospital with his hand on the door of the coffee shop and responded to my suggestion that he leave the muscle in place and do a modified rather than a radical on my patient by saying, "What difference does it make whether I do a radical or a modified radical? The breast is gone anyway!" He then turned his back and abruptly closed the door after him.

I was flabbergasted. He seemed to be saying, "Once the breast is gone, she isn't a real woman anymore!" What difference can it possibly make if she has a nearly skeletonized chest or a nice muscle pad over the bone? The sexism in his statement was shocking. He obviously felt that if a woman lost a breast, she wasn't desirable anymore, so why be concerned about how her scarred chest looked (or how physically comfortable she was).

Another of my patients, who had had a modified mastectomy eleven years before, developed a new cancer in her other breast. She wanted a lumpectomy, but almost every surgeon I consulted was ready to do an old-fashioned Halsted. "Why are you so concerned about her second breast?"

the surgeons asked. They seemed to think that having lost one breast, the loss of a second breast was unimportant. The patient, on the other hand, valued her remaining breast; it was still a source of sexual pleasure to her. In fact, she thought that the loss of her second breast would be more devastating than her original operation. (She got her lumpectomy.)

Today researchers and clinicians alike feel that the real hope for curing breast cancer lies in some type of drug treatment. Two basic approaches—*chemotherapy* and *hormonal therapy*—are currently the major means of altering the environment of the cancer cells, thereby decreasing their growth rate and spread.

CHEMOTHERAPY

Powerful drugs are emerging as front-line weapons against cancer. More than fifty potent cytotoxic (cell-killing) chemicals—used individually or in combination—are being given experimentally to attack and kill malignant cells. One day drugs may be used as the first line of defense against breast cancer, without surgery or radiation. Today, however, this is not possible.

Currently, cytotoxic drugs are used and are beneficial in treating extensive breast cancer, metastatic breast cancer, and cancer that has recurred after surgery. Extensive clinical trials are underway to evaluate the use of preventive adjuvant chemotherapy after surgery to rid the body of any small clusters of tumor cells lurking unnoticed. There is evidence that immediate postoperative therapy may be beneficial to women whose breast cancer has spread to their lymph nodes or beyond. (Preventive chemotherapy should not be used on women whose cancer is confined to the breast and has not spread to the lymph nodes because it has not been shown to offer benefit. It also carries risk.) Future trials may combine preventive chemotherapy with hormonal therapy or antiprostaglandin medications.

Some of the chemotherapy drugs most commonly used for breast cancer are methotrexate, cyclophosphamide, doxorubicin (adriamycin), 5-fluorouracil, thiotepa, phenylalanine mustard (L-PAN), chlorambucil, and vincristine. These various drugs have different mechanisms of action. Some have been used alone, but most physicians now tend to use combinations of several drugs to make sure that cancer cells are attacked during all their various phases of growth, thus increasing the chances of killing the tumor altogether. Currently it is possible to cause tumors to shrink in 50 to 75 percent of patients treated with one of many possible drug combinations.

All these chemotherapy drugs, however, are potentially dangerous, because they exert their toxic effects on all actively dividing cells, not only cancer cells. Therefore, they tend to produce major side effects such as decreases in red and white blood cell counts, bleeding problems, nausea, vomiting, fatigue, and hair loss. These problems are relieved when the drugs are discontinued or decreased in dosage. In combination, the drugs bring more complete remissions, often with side effects no greater than the side effects of each drug alone.

HORMONE MANIPULATION

Some metastatic breast cancers can best be treated by manipulating the body's hormones, either through surgery or medication. We know that some breast tumors are very dependent upon estrogen for their growth. These tumors contain "receptors" for estrogen. The more estrogen receptors the tumor has, the more dependent it is likely to be and the more easily it may respond to hormonal therapy.

Until recently, surgery has been used to deprive the body of estrogen by removing the ovaries, adrenals, or pituitary. (The pituitary produces no estrogen itself but directs the activity of the ovary and adrenal.) Paradoxically, postmenopausal women have also been treated medically by giving them large doses of estrogen, which may slow tumor growth in women long deprived of estrogen. Others have been treated with male hormone to shrink their tumors.

Hormone therapy may be combined with chemotherapy to increase the benefits of treatment. For example, an antiestrogen drug could deny estrogen to the tumor cells that need it to grow and divide; a cell-killing (cytotoxic) drug then can attack the weakened cancer cells. The results of the combined treatment are better than either drug alone could produce.

By far the most exciting news in hormonal therapy for breast metastases is a drug called Novaldex (tamoxifen citrate), an antiestrogen medication that vies with estrogen for the estrogen-receptor sites. Once the drug "uses up" these sites, estrogen can no longer attach to the cell. The cell then loses the ability to grow and reproduce itself. When this happens, the cancer cells die and the tumor shrinks.

For several years, Novaldex has been considered the preferred means of producing hormonal change for postmenopausal patients with advanced breast cancer, and recently it has been used to treat premenopausal women. It can save women from major surgery to remove their ovaries, which are still producing the estrogen that encourages tumor growth. Because Novaldex is an antiestrogen and not a hormone or a cytotoxic agent, the adverse reactions commonly associated with these types of drugs in cancer therapy are avoided or minimized. There have been no reports of liver, kidney, or cardiac damage associated with Novaldex therapy. While most patients have no or few side effects, some patients experience slight hot flashes, nausea, vomiting; or unpredictable increases in blood-calcium levels may occur in patients with bony metastases. This side effect is rare but can be severe if it occurs. On the positive side, the drug is given twice a day in pill form, so that hospitalization is not necessary for treatment.

Clinical results show that 61 percent of postmenopausal patients derive benefits from Novaldex therapy. Four percent achieve complete remission, 35 percent partial remission, 22 percent stabilization, and 39 percent fail to respond.

These early test results suggest that the response to this drug is as good as the response to surgery (removal of the ovaries). Research is also underway on a new drug, aminglutethimide, which suppresses the adrenal gland's production of sex steroid and probably inhibits the production of tumor-nurturing estrogen in the body fat. The adrenal glands, like the estrogen-producing ovaries, are often removed from women with growing tumors; but if this new drug works, adrenalectomy will no longer be necessary. Drugs such as tamoxifen and aminglutethimide may soon make it possible to avoid some major surgical procedures that have been part of the routine health care of women with metastatic disease. To me, that's awfully good news.

Novaldex is an antiestrogen, but interestingly enough, the drug also has antiprostaglandin properties. Recent evidence has suggested that prostaglandins may play a part in tumor spread and growth in bones, and that drugs that inhibit prostaglandins may be valuable therapeutic agents in treating cancer, particularly breast cancer that has spread to bone. Studies are underway in Europe, and soon will be in the United States, in which women with bony metastases are given other antiprostaglandin drugs, alone or in addition to their usual chemotherapy. Because they have minimal side effects, these drugs will be a welcome addition to the usual options for women with advanced breast cancer.

One of my patients who had a radical mastectomy eleven years ago did well for nearly ten years, but then began to have severe pain in her back. After an orthopedist had been treating her "for arthritis" for some time, she decided to return to see me. Unfortunately, by that time, her original breast cancer had spread widely throughout her bones and she was nearly unable to walk and was constantly on narcotics for pain.

I hospitalized her in order to determine the extent of her disease, to give her some rest and pain relief, and to give her radiation therapy to decrease some of the bone pain. The chemotherapists at the hospital decided that she should be placed on their usual multidrug regimen for metastatic breast cancer, but I was adamantly opposed. I felt that my patient had developed her breast cancer in an estrogen milieu. I did not think that estrogen had caused her breast cancer, but the estrogen she had received during ten years of taking birth-control pills and four years of estrogen-replacement therapy had been part of her total body chemistry during the formative years of the tumor. In this estrogen-enriched environment, the tumor had grown.

Since estrogen-receptor sites were unknown at the time of my patient's breast surgery eleven years before, it was not possible to determine that she actually had such sites. Nevertheless, I felt strongly that her tumor must have been estrogen-site positive because of her high hormonal intake and long period of survival. So I refused to allow the chemotherapists' choice of treatment. My patient and I talked at great length about the choice of an antiestrogen drug. Novaldex was just becoming known in breast-cancer work, and both of us decided it was worth a go.

Novaldex was a good choice for her. Within a few weeks, she was up and walking, first with a walker, then with a cane, and as her pain completely subsided, she gave up her cane. For the past year and a half, she has led a normal life. She drives, cooks, shops, and feels fine. She has no side effects that I can determine—no hair loss, no nausea, no weight loss, and no anemia. In fact, she appears to be normal in every way, except for her mastectomy scar. As scientific documentation of her progress, her bone scan, which originally showed multiple areas of metastatic cancer spread to bone, has now returned to normal.

Such a feat was impossible, even unthinkable, five years ago. Five years ago, this patient would have been dead within two to three months of her radiation therapy. I also am convinced that she would have died if she had gotten the usual chemotherapy.

Some ten years ago, I had another patient who had breast cancer and also developed metastases to her bones. She was in her early sixties. She was hospitalized for a fracture of the hip resulting from the bony metastasis. I had taken a Pap smear and estrogen-level count the week before she went into the hospital. The medical technician read her slides and showed me the results. This patient had an extraordinarily high amount of estrogen in her body—most unusual for a woman over 60. Although postmenopausal women are quite often treated with estrogen for metastatic disease, I immediately felt that just adding the usual estrogen to this woman's already abnormally high amounts of circulating estrogen would not benefit her in any way. So, instead, I gave her male hormone. Her bone pain improved, and she was able to be up and about and to take care of her grandson for nearly two years. If Novaldex had been available at that time, she might have lived even longer.

I only bring this case up because, as far as I know, estrogen levels are never considered when deciding on the treatment of women with metastatic breast cancer. Perhaps in those cases where surgery was done years ago, when no tests for estrogen-receptor sites were done, and where none can be obtained at the present time, doctors should do a simple estrogen-level test. It may not prove anything, but if the estrogen level is elevated, it could be a clue that hormonal therapy is indicated. The procedure is as simple as taking a Pap. I currently follow all my breast-cancer patients with estrogen-level tests every six months. I am not sure what may be proved, but any significant change in their levels would make me suspicious that all was not well. These women are, of course, also followed up with blood tests, bone scans, and chest X-rays. The estrogen level provides another piece of information that one day might turn out to be of value.

It is unpleasant but accurate to say that women are being used as guinea pigs every day. Because doctors do not know what surgical procedure or chemotherapy is best, in participating centers women with breast cancer who consent to be studied are assigned randomly to different treatments. Depending on chance, they will have a modified radical or a lumpectomy followed by radiation. Doctors will monitor their progress, count the statistics, and hope to make the world a little better for future victims of breast cancer. The same procedure is used with chemotherapy for women who develop metastatic disease. Various hospitals around the country are trying different set regimens of drugs. Their results and follow-up studies on patients will be sent into a national program, where the mortality and morbidity figures will be tallied and recommendations will be made for continuing the use of certain drugs, discontinuing the use of other drugs, and combining drugs.

Hopefully, progress will come from these studies. However, sometimes these rigid research protocols cloud the issue for an individual patient. Remember my patient who would have been placed on the hospital's usual chemotherapy regimen rather than the Novaldex that I wanted her to receive? In addition, the type of breast surgery or nonsurgery you receive may depend simply upon where you live. For example, if you have a cancer of the breast and you live in New York and go to Memorial Hospital, you will be more likely to have a radical mastectomy. On the other hand, if you live in Boston, you may not have surgery but will be more likely to undergo radiation. In other words, your treatment may depend more on the practice characteristics of an area than on the particular character of your disease.

One of the obvious problems with breast cancer is that often the disease spreads early. This is why it is so important that women learn to practice BSE rigorously and to take advantage of the new early-detection techniques. But another obvious problem is that many doctors are all too willing to perform unnecessary, outdated radical procedures. Recent cancer research has produced good news about early detection and minimal surgery. Now it's up to women who have Stage I or Stage II cancer to insist upon these appropriate lesser procedures. Sometimes it seems that the intimidated female cancer patient, faced by her surgeon, loses her nerve; but I am convinced that, given the information we need, we have all the stamina that may be required to insist on proper treatment.

One of my patients, whom I'll call Gloria, recently went to the hospital for an outpatient breast biopsy, after denying the surgeon her consent to a one-step biopsy-and-mastectomy procedure. She had a 9 A.M. operating-room appointment, and I met her afterward at a noon luncheon. She was wearing an enormous smile, so I immediately knew her biopsy had proven the tumor to be benign.

"You look great," I said. "Do you have any discomfort?"

She shook her head and said, "I don't even need an aspirin." She grinned at me as she continued, "I must tell you about this morning. The surgeon injected a little Novocain and began to remove the lump. He kept peeking up at my face, which was behind a little piece of sheet, and saying, "Are you all right?" Finally I couldn't stand his anxiety anymore, so when he asked me again, I said, "Yes, doctor, I'm fine. As a matter of fact, I'm doing better than you are."

And so could we all, if we would put our fears behind us, take advantage of new techniques, and act in our own best interests.

CHAPTER 5

No More Hot Flashes: Menopause and Estrogen-Replacement Therapy

Having triumphed over dysmenorrhea and breast cancer, we can now look forward to menopause! The menopausal woman is a twentieth-century phenomenon. In the fourteenth century, a woman's average life expectancy was 33 years. At the turn of this century, it had increased to 48 years, and older women were not yet a "problem," as they simply didn't exist in significant numbers. The life expectancy of a woman born today, however, is 77.3 years. Menopause has become the midpoint of a woman's life, not the impending end.[1] Today, women can count on spending much of their lives in the postmenopausal state.

In the human female, the ovaries die before their owner. And the loss of ovarian function that occurs at menopause deprives the woman not just of fertility, but also of important female hormones produced by the ovary. While medical science cannot restore a menopausal woman's fertility, it can replace her hormones.

In many different types of glandular failure, modern medicine can replace hormones. For example, if the thyroid fails, replacement therapy is given and continued indefinitely. Likewise, failure of the adrenal and the pancreas are similarly treated. However, until the 1960s, it was considered a natural event when the ovaries failed, and the patient was usually advised not to interfere with nature. Menopause was considered natural, desirable, and even good for our health. Many menopausal women, however, endured a variety of complaints—erratic menstruation, sudden blood-vessel changes producing hot flashes and night sweats, anxiety, and depression.

The intensity of the menopausal symptoms a woman suffers depends on several factors. At menopause, a woman does not suddenly lose 100 percent of her estrogen. The ovarian tissue still produces small amounts of estrogen. The adrenal and the ovary also produce a weak male hormone, androstenedione, part of which becomes converted by the body's fat into estrogen. As the ovary decreases its output of estrogen, its production of androstenedione remains relatively static. This creates a change in the relative proportions of male and female hormones, and in turn, results in subtle changes that cause the appearance of dark, coarse facial hairs on the chin and also possibly some arteriosclerotic problems.

It is clear that there is marked individual variation in the amount and proportion of the remaining hormones the ovaries produce, as well as in the total length of time that this occurs. This is why some women have severe symptoms, while others have few complaints. Women with more fat tend to be able to convert more androstenedione to estrogen and have fewer symptoms. Some women may never become symptomatic: they may produce hormones over a longer period of time and have a slower waning of the entire process.

The worst suffering occurs in women who suddenly lose their functioning ovaries through surgery or radiation. Because of the abruptness of the estrogen loss, the hot flashes, irritability, and anxiety that ensue are often intolerable. For most women, however, the estrogen loss occurs at a moderate rate. The symptoms these women experience are milder. The total effect of the loss of estrogen depends, in large measure, on your own genetic resistance to aging, your overall health, quality of diet, and activity.

During the 1950s, women were treated for these symptoms

with vitamin and exercise programs and tranquilizers, but by the 1960s, doctors were attributing all menopausal symptoms to lost estrogen and enthusiastically offering to put it back. Estrogen-Replacement Therapy (ERT) became standard treatment for menopausal symptoms.

My first acquaintance with ERT came when I, as a new doctor just out of medical school, was making house calls with my senior partner. We were let into a thoroughly messy apartment by a disheveled, middle-aged woman in a bathrobe. She told us that she couldn't cope any longer. She was extremely depressed, and her whole life seemed to be made worse by her constant hot flashes. My associate, Florence, gave her an injection and a few pills. When we got back into the car, I asked,

"What did you give her?"

"A shot of estrogen and some estrogen pills."

This was my first experience with estrogen therapy. It had never been taught in medical school.

Some ten days later, I was working in the office when I noticed a patient I had never seen before sitting in the waiting room. She was pretty, neatly dressed and made up; she sat there smiling, with her gloved hands calmly folded in her lap.

"Who is that?" I asked Florence.

"Don't you recognize her? That's the woman we gave the estrogen to on our house call."

I was flabbergasted. Seeing the remarkable transformation in that woman made an indelible impression on me, and in 1964, I began to use ERT rather freely for patients with hot flashes and night sweats.

Then, in the mid-seventies, the media began to report higher than normal rates of endometrial (uterine) cancer in women who had been on ERT. Everywhere frightened women stopped their therapy. Among my own patients, many decided to grit their teeth and endure hot flashes rather than risk the hypothetical development of uterine cancer. (Of course, many women in this age group have had hysterectomies, and if you have no uterus, you don't have to worry about uterine cancer.)

As the controversy went on, I thought that I had some important evidence to offer, for my patients had been treated differently all along. Since the ovaries produce *two* female hormones, estrogen and progesterone, it had always seemed to me to be just plain common sense that if I was going to replace one of them, I should replace the other as well. If nature had found it necessary to provide both, I, a mere physician, was not going to presume to improve upon that. It seemed to me that, even in the cycle of posthysterectomy patients who had no uterus, the progesterone was essential to counteract the effects of the estrogen on the breasts. Therefore, each of my ERT patients received estrogen plus a monthly injection of progesterone or progesterone in the form of Provera tablets.

Often, my patients were puzzled. Taking progesterone in addition to the estrogen gave them back the full cycle each month, complete with menstruation. Why, they wanted to know, did they need this method, when all their friends who went to other doctors got only estrogen. Their friends never got their periods back, or if they did, their doctors did an immediate D & C. So along with their medication, each one of my patients got a long discussion on why I felt that progesterone had to be coupled with estrogen-replacement therapy.

When a young woman is cycling normally, her ovaries produce estrogen in the beginning of the cycle, and after she ovulates, they also produce progesterone. At the end of the cycle, both hormone levels fall, bringing about a complete shedding of the endometrial lining (menstruation).

The woman who does not ovulate does not produce progesterone, although she produces estrogen. Without progesterone, the endometrial lining of the uterus is constantly stimulated by estrogen. The lining grows and grows, and finally the thickened lining outgrows its blood supply. Then it begins to disintegrate haphazardly, a little from one spot, then a little from another. Because the lining is too thick to begin with, the flow is heavy. The flow is sporadic, too, and occurs over an extended period of time as one section after another sloughs off. This overgrowth of the lining, stimulated by estrogen, is similar to the hyperplasia, or cell overcrowding, which is sometimes thought to be an precursor of endometrial cancer.

On the other hand, when ovulation occurs, the endometrial lining, developed normally under the influence of progesterone during the latter part of the cycle, is better differentiated and not crowded. When menstruation begins in an ovulatory cycle (or with progesterone added), in a few days, the lining cleanly and precisely sloughs off down to the normal base. No prolonged heavy flow here with days of irregular bleeding. Progesterone is a good housekeeper. It efficiently gets rid of all the old, useless cells and prepares for the new month.

Most physicians, recognizing the danger of too much estrogen stimulation, tell their patients to take estrogen for only three weeks of each month. But a study by Dr. Kupperman of the New York University Medical Center demonstrated that when the patient stops taking estrogen for a week, her body fat releases estrogen it has stored, so the effect of estrogen continues.[2] It's not just the periodic break from added estrogen that women need; it's progesterone.

On the whole, my patients didn't mind getting their periods back. Few of them were overjoyed, but when they understood that this was a safer way to replace their hormones—since it was nature's way—they accepted it. The menses that occurred were pain-free, and most were over in two to four days. Patients who were on 0.625 milligram or smaller doses of estrogen often had no more than a day of spotting, because they did not receive sufficient estrogen to build up enough lining to create a heavier flow. With the use of smaller doses in older patients, no flow occurs.

One of the questions that my patients always asked was,

"Doctor, if I get my periods back, can I get pregnant?" The answer is a definite no! Doctors can replace the hormones that the ovaries are no longer capable of producing, but we are not smart enough to be able to cause the shriveled ovaries to rejuvenate themselves and to produce eggs again.

In 1976, when I gave my speech to the conference on working women, the media were just beginning their exposé of ERT as a cause of uterine cancer. I knew that estrogen-replacement therapy without progesterone was bound to cause problems, and, in fact, women who were on ERT without progesterone might well be better off without their therapy. So when I gave my speech, I argued that estrogen should not be given alone.

I feel that it is the misuse of estrogen, and not the estrogen per se, that is the culprit and the cause of the prevailing controversy. If the basis of endometrial carcinoma lies in the progression from endometrial hyperplasia to cystic hyperplasia to adenomatous hyperplasia to adenocarcinoma, then the physician who misuses estrogen is at fault. He is not providing natural ovarian replacement because he is leaving out progesterone, which would not permit even the first step in the sequence, i.e. hyperplasia, to occur.

The male-dominated ob/gyn ranks have for the most part never bothered to add progesterone to the woman's regimen because adding progesterone causes a menstrual flow each month, and this is too much fuss for the doctor or the patient to deal with. Because of this attitude estrogen has been used alone. The uterine lining, therefore, is continuously stimulated by the estrogen without the relief afforded by the antiestrogen effect of progesterone. By adding progesterone, the cells lining the uterine cavity are sloughed off each month. They are not allowed to sit around, get old, and into trouble. The woman gets a clean bill of health each month as fresh new cells replace the old.

Estrogen should not be given without progesterone. If we are truly doing replacement therapy, then we must replace both hormones produced by the ovary, not just the estrogen alone.[3]

The menopausal woman has reached a plateau in her life.

She may be reentering the job market, prepared to devote her energy to work now that her domestic chores are behind her. As she begins her new life, she finds that her menstrual periods have gotten somewhat irregular, and she begins to be bombarded by hot flashes. She wakes up two to three times a night in a pool of sweat. She changes her nightgown, changes her bed, and goes back to sleep as best she can. She is in a very peculiar mental state. She's not quite sure what the matter is. Things are going well, life with her husband is good. Money is no problem, maybe for the first time in their lives. She's working, the kids are established and, yet, she feels depressed. She feels blue and cries.

Some women never have this experience. Some women never experience a menstrual cramp or throw up during pregnancy. Likewise, some women don't do well through their menopause. Some doctors will tell you that women who are weak and who have problems will have a very bad menopause, but stable women won't. I say, "Bunk." From observing the very healthy, intellectual, and intelligent group of menopausal women that I see in my practice, I believe that the physical changes that occur in menopause affect the mental outlook of these women. Upon careful questioning, they will say they're usually aware of some degree of depression and of increasing emotional swings.

The aging process in women is distorted by the loss of the ovarian function. Menopause blends insidiously into the process of aging. The distinct symptoms of menopause are often confused with the general symptoms of aging, presenting a confused picture to the physician, which he often chooses not to treat.[4]

But I was not willing to throw out ERT. As far as I was concerned, the media had based their scare headlines on terribly misleading studies, for none of them documented cases of women who had received both estrogen and progesterone. All across the country, most women on ERT had received only estrogen, but I had in my practice many women who not only had been on combined estrogen-progesterone therapy, but had been on it for years. So I began several years ago to identify all the patients in my practice who had been on ERT with progesterone for 6 months or more. I counted 74 patients who had received estrogen every day for 6 to 150 months—cycled with progesterone—for meno-pausal symptoms including hot flashes, night sweats, atrophic vaginitis, depression, and/or patient complaints of person-ality changes, such as the inability to "think straight" or to function as before. With the help of a well-known pa-thologist[5] and the computer math department at the State University at Stony Brook, I did a retrospective study of those patients and compared them to a group of 473 women in my practice who were not on ERT. The study was pub-lished in the *Journal of Reproductive Medicine* in May 1979.[6]

A computer analysis of the data from my study revealed that the 74 patients who were on long-term estrogen-pro-gesterone therapy had tended to lose weight during the time they were on therapy. I concluded that the weight loss was probably due to their being examined and weighed on a regular basis and my habit of encouraging my patients to stay trim, rather than the consequence of the estrogen-pro-gesterone regimen.

Blood pressure, blood sugars, and cholesterol levels re-mained unchanged in these women. Pap smears, however, tended to improve. Nine patients had a Pap class improve-ment in their Pap smears (Class II to Class I), while two had some worsening (one, Class I to Class II; one, Class II to Class III) (see page 245 for an explanation of these classifications).

The most exciting part of the study was determining what changes had taken place within the uteri of the women who had been on long-term therapy. Decent office aspiration (suc-tion) methods first became available three years before the study ended, and I performed biopsies on 25 of the 74 treated patients. (For various medical or personal reasons, the remaining 48 patients could not be biopsied; 15 had undergone hysterectomies prior to going on ERT and be-coming my patients, 2 could not be biopsied because the opening into the uterus was too small, and 32 either refused aspiration, had moved from the area, or were no longer on therapy at the time the aspirations were being performed.) The average duration of estrogen-progesterone therapy at the time of the biopsy was 57.2 months (4.9 years), with a range of from 6 to 150 months. For comparison, 28 women over 40 who were part of the 473-patient control group were also biopsied.

Interestingly, most of the uterine biopsies of the ERT patients did not reflect that they had received continuous estrogen. The most common finding (in 10 patients) was a normal secretory endometrium resulting from progesterone. This indicates the important conclusion that progesterone, in sufficient quantity, counteracts, supersedes, and modifies the estrogen effect even when estrogen is given on a continual daily basis over long periods of time.

The next most common finding (in 8 patients) was an inactive endometrium. These uterine linings show no indications that they had responded either to estrogen or to progesterone; the uterine linings simply had lost all function and could not be rejuvenated.

Five others showed normal early cycle endometrium (proliferative endometrium). There were also two cases of hyperplasia, one slight, one adenomatous. Their therapy was changed and six months later when they were biopsied again, both endometria had become inactive. (One patient was placed on a lower dose of estrogen and took her usual progesterone, the other patient was placed on progesterone therapy without estrogen.)

Among the control group, none had received estrogen-progesterone therapy, but the statistical comparisons of the results of the endometrial aspiration biopsies performed on the 25 ERT patients and the 28 controls showed no significant differences, even though there was a case of uterine cancer among the controls. After studying the data from this tiny but probably representative sample, I concluded my report by saying that "the use of long-term estrogen does not necessarily lead inevitably to hyperplasia, cystic hyperplasia, adenomatous hyperplasia, and adenocarcinoma"—all of which are technical terms for progressive stages we believe lead to cancer (see pages 230–36). "It is reasonable to assume that the first step of the sequence is eliminated by the use of a progesterone in sufficient dosage. It is, therefore, suggested that problems encountered with the use of estrogen in menopausal patients can be averted by cycling these patients with progesterone."

Because the number of patients in my study was small, no definitive conclusions should be drawn from the data, but these same trends were confirmed by another, much larger retrospective study published by Dr. Hammond and his associates in the *American Journal of Obstetrics/Gynecology,* March 1, 1979. Two groups of women were analyzed. Both were deficient in estrogen because of surgical removal of their ovaries, menopause, or some other reason. One group of 301 women was treated with estrogen; the other group of 309 was not. Long-term estrogen therapy (for more than five years) resulted in "significantly lower rates of development of cardiovascular disease, hypertension, osteoporosis, and fractures." It was also noted that the women on estrogen took much less medication in the categories of tranquilizers and sedatives. There was a significant reduction in the new occurrences of strokes, coronary artery disease, congestive heart failure, and arteriosclerotic cerebral vascular disease, and a "lower incidence of weight gain."[7]

Hammond showed, however, that the women who were cycled on estrogen *alone* had an increased incidence of endometrial cancer. There were only three cases of endometrial cancer among the nontreated control group of women, as opposed to eleven cases in the group treated with estrogen only. Among the one-quarter of the treated group who received estrogen and progesterone, there were no endometrial cancers at all. That led him to conclude that there was actually a reduction of incidence of malignancy over that which would occur naturally in the group of women who took progesterone along with estrogen.

Similar results were reported in a study by Dr. R. D. Gambrell in the October 1978 *Southern Medical Journal.* Among 1,694 patients receiving estrogen alone, he found the incidence of endometrial cancer to be 3.5 per 1,000. For the estrogen-progesterone users, the incidence was 0.4 per

1,000, a rate *lower* than the spontaneous occurrence of endometrial malignancy in untreated postmenopausal women.

More evidence in favor of using progesterone along with estrogen comes from studies of young women who have abnormal genes and ovaries that do not function correctly. A woman with polycystic ovaries, for example, does not ovulate; the endometrium is constantly stimulated by estrogen alone without the relief provided by progesterone. Since a woman with this condition does not ovulate, she cannot get pregnant, which also deprives her of an arrest to the growth of the uterine lining for nine months. These women are genetically unstable and have a continuous growth stimulation from their own estrogen. Based on those criteria, it is expected that they would be more prone to cancer of the uterus, and they are.

Despite all this evidence, I am convinced that the final answer to the ERT controversy will not be found for at least ten years. It will take that long for truly scientific large-scale studies to clarify the subject.

In the meantime, simply backing off from ERT for fear of uterine cancer seems to me to be a mistake. For one thing, the role of estrogen in stimulating uterine cancer is far from clear. Although the thickened uterine lining that develops in patients on estrogen therapy without progesterone resembles the first stage leading to cancer, there seems to be a second, later stage of development that does not depend upon estrogen. In fact, this second stage may result from a temporary lapse in hormones controlling cell growth.

These days, a lot of physicians speculate about whether women who take estrogen and subsequently get endometrial cancer really have "regular endometrial cancer." More often than not, the type of uterine cancer women on therapy develop is not as invasive and malignant as that of women who are not on therapy. Most of the uterine cancers seen in women on estrogen are early cancers that are confined to the uterus and have not spread beyond its borders.

In addition, doctors point out that there are many other

factors besides estrogen that contribute to the development of cancer. Genetic predisposition is only one example. We hear more and more about "cancer families," and indeed, many women who develop uterine cancer have family histories of uterine endometrial cancer or gastrointestinal cancer. They also seem to share certain traits. They tend to be big-boned or obese and to have hypertension or diabetes. They also tend to have heavy menses and late menopause. In addition, most women who develop uterine cancer tend to belong to the upper economic class, to marry late or remain single, to be sterile or have few pregnancies, and to be white.

As far as I can determine, estrogen therapy has never been proven to cause breast cancer. Estrogen is not a carcinogen. In fact, no known natural hormone has been proved to be a cause of human cancer. Estrogen is a growth stimulant,* however, so it can stimulate an already-present breast cancer to grow.

Just before this book went to press, there was an article by Ross et al. in *JAMA (Journal of the American Medical Association).*[8] It reviewed the incidence of breast cancer in women treated with ERT versus a control group in two retirement communities. The study was retrospective. Here, as in nearly all other studies, the women were treated with estrogen and *without progesterone.* The researchers found a statistically significant increase in breast cancer in women receiving ERT who had intact ovaries, but not in those women whose ovaries had been removed. There was no increase in those women who had received low-dose estrogen. Further, for those women who had their ovaries removed, there was a slight, but not statistically significant, decrease in breast cancer associated with ERT.

The results of this study are confusing as well as disturbing. Uterine cancer, I feel, can be anticipated and dealt with, but breast cancer is a much more serious matter. Drs. Meier

---

*Other growth stimulants include growth hormone, thyroid hormone, and protein.

and Landau wrote an editorial in the same issue of *JAMA*[9] and stated that the estrogen doses in the above study were higher than would currently be prescribed by "thoughtful" physicians. They also stated that "the overall results do not show a significant difference in estrogen use between cases and controls."

I am sure that many more studies will soon be coming forth to help shed light on this subject. As of this time, the question is still very much unsettled. This problem needs and deserves the fullest attention and support of the research community.

So the cancer risks from ERT are by no means clear-cut. But on the other side of the coin there are some positive benefits to be gained from ERT with progesterone. Before I go on to discuss those benefits, however, I must point out that there are some specific contraindications to using ERT. If you have any of these conditions, you definitely should not consider ERT, with or without progesterone.

breast cancer
uterine cancer or undiagnosed vaginal bleeding
known or suspected pregnancy
past history of active thrombophlebitis (blood clots)

The following are relative contraindications. Women who have these conditions may take estrogen, but must be closely monitored.

migraine headaches
liver disease
seizure disorders (epilepsy)
hypertension
fibrocystic disease of the breast
connective tissue disease
family history of high blood fat levels
diabetes
gall-bladder disease
multiple sclerosis

What little we know of genetic predisposition to cancer suggests that women should be carefully screened before they are given estrogen. Women who have had a hysterectomy for a reason other than cancer should have less fear of estrogen therapy; but among women who still have the uterus, those who, as mentioned before, are large-boned, obese, hypertensive, and/or diabetic probably should not start on estrogen unless they are carefully followed by their physician. In every case, a Pap, a mammography, blood work, and an endometrial biopsy must be done before initiating estrogen therapy. And any woman who goes on ERT should be seen by her physician every six months.

But what about the benefits of ERT? Should you consider it? Is it good for you?

Most women begin ERT treatment to alleviate symptoms such as hot flashes and night sweats, which are simply episodes of hot flashes that occur during the sleeping hours. Hot flashes are uncomfortable enough during the waking hours, but night sweats can cause additional problems by interfering with sleep. Women complain that they either can't fall asleep or can't sleep through the night. Women who suffer night sweats feel tired, weak, and unable to function. Sleep deprivation can make anyone feel depressed and chronically out of sorts.

Recent studies have shown that women on ERT sleep better and fall asleep faster, but such symptomatic relief may not get at all the underlying problems. Although there are some 30 to 40 million postmenopausal women in the United Sates, three-quarters of whom experience hot flashes, very little research has been done on the cause of this problem. This oversight is unfortunate but, perhaps, predictable in view of the medical profession's customary inattention to "female complaints." We do know, however, that the hot flashes are *real.* Many women have been told that they are imagined or made worse by their state of mind, but actual recordings of skin temperature in the fingers show that there are large increases in skin temperature that correlate closely with the complaints of hot flashes.[10] There is also evidence that the hot flashes are accompanied by dramatic increases in LH, a pituitary hormone.[11] Hot flashes, therefore, are associated with hormonal disturbances in the hypothalamus, the heat-regulatory center of the brain. They are not symptoms dreamed up by women who have nothing better to do than complain.

Nevertheless, as with dysmenorrhea, male physicians intimate that if menopausal women could just get it all together, their hot flashes would go away. They often prescribe tranquilizers to treat hot flashes, although such drugs don't answer the specific problem. Sedation is not the answer to physiologic symptoms, yet women are customarily sedated with tranquilizers for almost any complaint they voice. Like dysmenorrhea, hot flashes have a real cause, and a scientific treatment should be prescribed. It is time to put the onus back on the doctors, who, because they don't know the answers, make us feel inadequate and guilty, and then put us under sedation. It is efficient, however, for prescribing a tranquilizer gets rid of the patient and clears the waiting room.

In controlling hot flashes, estrogen is very effective, while substitutes like the progestogen Provera or Depo-Provera are somewhat less so. New medications like Catapres (Boehringer-Ingelheim Corp.) or Propranolol (Inderal-Ayerst Labs), both antihypertensives with many side effects, show some promise. But menopause involves more than the hot flash. Concentrating on the hot flash is like treating a pneumonia patient with only cough syrup. The syrup might get rid of the cough, but the patient is still sick from her infection. Catapres might get rid of hot flashes, but still leaves a woman with atrophic vaginitis, osteoporosis, and depression. It's necessary to consider a woman's overall condition. As a patient, you should try to make sure your doctor is considering all aspects of your menopausal experience.

The reaction of the medical profession to menopausal symptoms is interesting and somewhat dismaying to observe. One of the factors affecting whether some male physicians treat a woman with menopausal complaints is the presence of dyspareunia (painful intercourse). Physicians who will not treat such discomforts as hot flashes, night sweats, or insomnia will treat women with estrogen should they complain of pain and dryness during intercourse. Not only will they treat them with estrogen, but they will treat them forever for this condition.

Painful intercourse due to lack of estrogen usually begins to occur late in menopause and may be accompanied by vaginal dryness, tenderness, itching, and bleeding. Women with this condition become more prone to vaginal infection, because the wall of the vagina is becoming thinner and because there is a lessening of normal cleansing and protective secretions. The normal, younger vagina has some thirty cell layers and is a strong, well-lubricated organ. In late menopause, it thins down to as little as six cell layers because of estrogen deprivation.

But these aspects of vaginal aging do not seem to be the physician's chief concern. I had an interesting conversation with one of the world's foremost pharmacologists about this. I asked him whether he approved of treating postmenopausal women with estrogen. He smiled at me and said that he was not really in favor of therapy unless, of course, the woman was having dyspareunia. I smiled back and replied, "You mean that you feel that a woman should only receive estrogen when her symptoms interfere with a male function?" After a long silence, he smiled sheepishly and said, "Yes, I think that is correct." He confirmed something that I had always suspected. Our medical therapy really does get slanted by the male physician's whims and prejudices. It is not always what is good for us but what he believes our role should be that counts (especially when it affects his or another male's pleasure).

Male opinions aside, women who hope to continue an active sex life into their late fifties, sixties, and seventies may want to consider ERT. Estrogen will not make you young again, but it can have a profound effect on your vagina, which returns to its youthful state very quickly after estrogen-replacement therapy has begun and will maintain itself as long as replacement continues.

Urologic problems also occur in menopause, because the urinary tract, especially the lower portion, is situated close to the vagina, and its tissues are also dependent upon estrogen for their support. Some older women experience multiple, recurring bladder infections as these tissues become more fragile. Since estrogen may help build up the defenses of the bladder and urinary tract against bacteria, such infections may be reduced by adding estrogen to the usual antibiotic regimens. Menopausal women may also notice involuntary loss of urine upon coughing, sneezing, or running. Sometimes they are forced to wear a sanitary pad continuously. Some physicians prescribe corrective surgery for this complaint, but estrogen therapy in the form of estrogen creams, with or without estrogen by mouth, should be tried first if there are no contraindications.

Let me interject one additional note on estrogen creams while we are on the subject. Some women have been led to believe that they do not carry the same risks as oral estrogens. A recent study in the *Journal of the American Medical Association (JAMA)* shows that this is not so.[12] Two estrogen creams (Premarin and Estrace), when used vaginally, not only had local effects in the vagina but were well absorbed into the blood. Many women who currently use these products for vaginal dryness and itching should realize that long-term daily use of vaginal creams carries the same risks as taking estrogen orally.

Although ERT can bring relief from these common menopausal complaints, there are other reasons for ERT that are perhaps more important. They include changes in the bones, vagina, breasts, and vulva, and muscle weakness in the hip, back, and shoulders. Loss of bone density in the spine leads to backache and diminished height. The loss of height is caused by the vertebrae crushing and collapsing together. It is a common symptom among elderly women and accounts for the stereotyped image of the "little old lady."

Perhaps the most important reason to consider ERT is the prevention of osteoporosis, or brittle bones, one of the most neglected diseases of women. Because most women develop clinically significant osteoporosis within ten years of menopause, some physicians feel that every woman over 45 should be on ERT. The disease affects women nine times more often than men, and white women are more likely to develop the problem than black women.

Most women over the age of 65 shrink in height by some two inches and develop other symptoms of osteoporosis, including lumbar back pain, rounding of the upper back, and periodontal disease. Standard laboratory tests usually show normal results, but careful scrutiny of X-rays often reveals evidence of poor mineralization of the bone.

Thin, delicate white women need to be the most concerned with the development of osteoporosis. In youth and middle age, women and men suffer approximately the same number of fractures, but after menopause, the loss of the female hormone in women makes them more subject to osteoporosis and much more likely to suffer bone fractures. Older white males, of course, still have their male hormones to protect their bones.

Women with osteoporosis are likely to suffer hip fractures. And hip fractures are a major cause of death among older women. The National Center for Health Statistics estimated that of 184,000 hip fractures in the United States in 1975, more than 132,000 occurred in women. Furthermore, Dr. Gordon observed that "one-third of osteoporotic women who suffer hip fracture die within six months. Hip fracture is the cause of death in nearly 58,000 women each year, compared with about 2,300 endometrial cancer deaths annually." For that reason, Gordon advocates "life-long, very low-dose estrogen supplementation for nearly all post-menopausal women to avert the risk of osteoporosis and fracture-related mortality."[13]

Prevention of osteoporosis involves long-term estrogen-replacement therapy. We are no longer talking about the smallest amount of estrogen for the shortest period of time. Treating osteoporosis means estrogen at least for the first three to five years after menopause, when the replacement seems to have the maximum beneficial effect on bone maintenance. Lila Nachtigall, in a ten-year double-blind study involving eighty-four pairs of menopausal patients, demonstrated that estrogen virtually halts the loss of bone. Women in her study who took only a placebo showed progressive bone loss, and seven of them suffered fractures. Among the group who received estrogen and progesterone, there was little bone loss and no broken bones.[14]

These facts must make us reconsider the advice that women are currently getting about the dangers of estrogen. Estrogen-replacement therapy for bone preservation can be accomplished with as little as 0.3 or 0.625 milligram of conjugated estrogen daily (or other low-dose estrogen) combined with progesterone, and it will probably save more lives because of the decrease in fractures than it will cost due to uterine cancer. Now the estimated death rate from hip fracture is considerably greater than from endometrial cancer.

Nachtigall concluded her study by saying:

> Approximately one of four white women at the age of 60 will have spinal compression fractures associated with osteoporosis. One woman of five will fracture a hip by age 90, and one out of six of these women will die within three months of their injury. It is clear that as life expectancy increases, osteoporosis may overshadow the currently debated aspects of the estrogen controversy, becoming the factor deserving the greater consideration.

It is possible that other factors aside from ERT can reduce bone loss and can be part of a revitalizing regimen. Exercise helps maintain bones in better metabolic shape. Sedentary women tend to have more osteoporosis than active ones.

So, if it is at all possible, get up and get out; walk and swim if you can. (I would not recommend that you try jogging unless you are already actively involved in the sport.) Adding calcium, Vitamin D, and fluoride to your daily vitamins will also help retard bone loss.

Recent studies suggest that Calcitonin (an experimental hormonelike drug) or stanozolol (Winstrol, an anabolic hormone) can benefit postmenopausal women with osteoporosis, though Winstrol tends to produce the masculinizing side effects of male hormones. Both of these treatments hold promise—especially for women with osteoporosis who cannot take estrogen because of previous cancer or some other reason—but for the average woman, I think the effects of estrogen are preferable.

Estrogen also seems to ward off arteriosclerosis. Younger women rarely have heart attacks. Since the rate of heart attack increases after the onset of menopause, when estrogen diminishes, there is some evidence that estrogen may have a protective effect against the occurrence of coronary artery disease. Some studies have shown that postmenopausal women have a decrease in their cholesterol levels after being treated with estrogen. A study by Dr. Barrett-Connor et al. (reported in *JAMA,* May 18, 1979) reviewed 1,496 women ranging in age from 55 to 74, of whom 39 percent were on ERT. The report states that lower cholesterol values were the most striking feature associated with ERT, particularly since an increase in cholesterol usually coincides with natural menopause. Other studies have shown that women on ERT experience a decline in the total cholesterol level and an increase in the level of High-Density Lipoproteins (HDLs), a substance which carries cholesterol out of the bloodstream and is thought to protect against atherosclerosis when it is present in high levels. Premenopausal women with high HDL levels have less coronary artery disease and fewer heart attacks than men of the same age, but with menopause and the loss of estrogen, HDL levels fall; the protection of HDL is lost, and accordingly, at menopausal age, a woman's chances of heart attack increase to a point equal to those of a man. If replacement doses of estrogen can keep the HDL levels up, this should be another indication in favor of ERT. And, as in the case of osteoporosis, the risk of death from cardiovascular disorder is greater than the risk of estrogen-induced endometrial cancer. The annual risk of estrogen-associated endometrial-cancer deaths is less than 1 per 1,000, while the risk of cardiovascular death after age 55 exceeds 10 per 1,000.

Emotional upsets may also come with the menopausal years. Menopause signifies not only the loss of fertility but the certainty of mortality and the knowledge that many dreams will never come true. The half-century mark is not always easy to face.

These fears of the middle-aged years strike men and women alike, but the menopausal woman often feels also that she has lost her femininity. Many doctors write that the depression and stresses that occur in the menopause stem from personality problems that have been present throughout the woman's life. If she is well put together, they imply, then the emotional stress of this period will be well handled. They feel that the fault lies totally with the inherent weakness in the woman's personality, and that estrogen certainly will have no benefit on emotions alone. It is possible that they are right, but I think otherwise.

I have seen profound personality changes in some patients who have begun ERT. Women who were crying and depressed, although previously they had been the backbone and strength of the family, suddenly rebounded on estrogen-replacement therapy as if by magic. I would estimate that over 70 percent of these women had a marked improvement.

I have been equally impressed by the problem that some of these women encountered when they went off estrogen. Several women actually had a recurrence of all their original emotional problems. Most, however, could be helped by either increasing their dose to 0.625 milligram of conjugated estrogen again or by weaning them off their estrogen slowly. These women were four to five years postmenopausal, yet the estrogen was still important to their psyches. This was many years after the "trauma" of menopause had passed, when adjustment to the postmenopausal state should have stabilized; yet some patients still felt remarkably better while taking estrogen and elected to maintain themselves either on small doses or on their normal dose.

They felt that the only other alternative would be tranquilizers, but most of my patients do not like to go about in a stupor, dazed to the point that they scarcely know what they are doing. We all know of the dangers of addiction and the side effects of tranquilizers and the toll they take every day on the lives of women. Yet many women who refuse estrogen become hooked on tranquilizers instead—which can be much more dangerous.

A patient came to me a year and a half ago because she desperately wanted to go on estrogen therapy. She already had seen four doctors, who had all refused to put her on it because they didn't believe in ERT. She explained that she was unable to sleep, that her arms itched continuously, that she had some hot flashes, but more importantly, that she wasn't functioning as well as she had six to eight months previously. She just couldn't seem to "get it all together," and because she was an accountant, her work was suffering. I said that while I approved of ERT, I couldn't prescribe it for her until she had been completely evaluated; that meant a Pap, an endometrial biopsy, and a mammography, as well as the usual blood-chemistry tests.

She had her tests, passed with flying colors, and was started on therapy. As is my schedule, I saw her every two weeks for three visits. Not only did she feel and look better, but a year and a half later, she still insists on her estrogen. She is convinced that it is estrogen that has restored her capacity to perform well. Is it her imagination?

Is there a placebo effect? Maybe, but it's the most convincing placebo I have ever come across. Too many women have told me the same story over the past fifteen years. All of them can't be wrong. ERT is not indicated for mental depression and neurosis. However, I think that if you do not feel well physically, you cannot do well mentally. Whether it's hot flashes, night sweats, or fatigue from improper hormone balances, you mind is weighed down by the problems of your body. When you feel tired or sick, your mind is burdened with your physical problems. In healthy people, the brain can operate freely.

Should you consider ERT? That depends. If after reading this chapter, you are still fearful, don't. If after reading this chapter, you want to take the smallest dose of estrogen for the smallest amount of time, do. If you have no symptoms of menopause and feel that you do not need ERT, that's fine. If you want estrogen forever because you are sedentary, thin, white, and fear for your bones, that's fine, too. You yourself must make these decisions. No doctor should ever criticize you because you will not take the estrogen that he thinks you should have, or because you want estrogen and he doesn't believe in ERT. Those decisions are personal and are yours, and only yours, to make. He must guide you, however, if there are contraindications to therapy. And if you do go on ERT, he must carefully monitor your progress.

Not all doctors do. I met a friend's aunt today. Hearing that I was writing a book on women's health, she immediately began lamenting the fact that her doctor had just taken away her estrogen. She had no energy, she said, and the hot flashes were terrible. "Why did he take you off your pills?" I asked.

"Because I started to bleed," she responded. She then quickly added, "But the bleeding has stopped, so everything must be all right."

"You mean that you didn't have an office aspiration or a D & C?"

"No, I had a Pap, though, but he just said to forget the whole thing."

"Did he have you on progesterone or suggest that you should take it now?"

"Progesterone—what's that?"

This was a typical example of a woman, given estrogen for years, without progesterone, having a bleeding episode for the first time. I'm not sure what the doctor was thinking, but if this woman has a malignancy, surely it will not go away by forgetting about it. She needed an endometrial biopsy to document what the cause of her bleeding was.

Women need better care. If physicians are going to give medication over a long period of time, then they must understand completely what they are doing—and so must the women who receive the therapy. Only then can the relative benefits and risks of specific therapies be accurately evaluated. This, indeed, is the art and the science of medicine.

This patient's doctor obviously did not understand the implications of her bleeding nor the necessity for an endometrial biopsy. A Pap smear is not sufficient to rule out endometrial pathology. ERT is a serious game, and doctors, above all, should be familiar with the rules.

The only additional advice I can give is that if you decide to take estrogen, insist upon the addition of progesterone. It can be in the form of 100 milligrams of progesterone in oil once a month as an injection into your buttock. It can be as Provera, 100 milligrams per month in the form of tablets, or Norlutate, 50 milligrams per month in the form of tablets. Or your doctor may suggest other progestogens. With such a regimen, you will have the benefits of ERT while avoiding the risks of endometrial overstimulation.

To recapitulate: estrogen-progesterone therapy may help prevent osteoporosis, vaginal atrophy and infection, bladder changes, coronary heart disease, hot flashes, and emotional disturbances. As for the risks, because of our ability to easily monitor patients on estrogen for uterine cancer I have less fear of uterine cancer than I have of broken bones and coronary artery disease. Uterine cancer is not as lethal.

If you begin estrogen-progesterone therapy for any reason, you do not have to fear the development of uterine cancer. If you use the natural sequence of estrogen and progesterone, and if you have a uterine biopsy before the beginning of therapy and every year after that, the possibility of your developing uterine cancer is extremely tiny, and possibly less than if you had no therapy at all.

But in any case, uterine cancer does not just sneak up and suddenly appear. It results from a process that can be watched over months and years. A three- to four-minute aspiration in your doctor's office every twelve months provides complete information on the status of your uterine lining. The endometrial biopsy, like the Pap smear, will give you plenty of warning if something needs to be attended to.

One other consideration may be cost, and you should know that the medical confusion regarding ERT carries over into the reimbursement policies of many medical-insurance companies. Some will not cover the cost of ERT because they consider it to be an unproven therapy, while others will not pay for it because they consider the symptoms being treated as "psychiatric disorders," which are often excluded from their coverage.

The decision whether Medicare and Medicaid will cover the cost of ERT in a given state is made by the medical review committee of the particular Medicare carrier or state Medicaid agency. These decisions vary from case to case and from season to season. The result is that the availability of the treatment for some women literally depends on the often biased perception of a few medical reviewers in an insurance or government office.

Again, the decisions you make do not have to be permanent. You may begin therapy and find that it is not all that you expected. Fine. Simply discontinue the treatment and inform your physician. You may also decide to seek the lowest possible dosage for the shortest possible amount of time. That, too, is fine. Take what you feel you must have and no more. If you want estrogen for three years or more, to keep your bones in the best possible condition, that's okay. But whatever you do, make sure you consider all the available facts. You know your mind and body better than anyone else. If you try estrogen-replacement therapy plus progesterone and it's good for you, continue. If it's not, stop. This decision, like any other, can be changed at any time. But remember, you may be spending a large part of your life as a postmenopausal woman. It is important that you make an informed, well-considered choice about what is best for your body and the quality of your life.

CHAPTER 6

Keeping Your Uterus and Keeping It Healthy

Sally's gynecologist had just given her her yearly physical examination. Dr. P. smiled at her and said, "Sally, your fibroids have grown a bit in the last year. Since you are 38 years old and have two children, I think it's time you had your hysterectomy. You'll be in the hospital a little over a week, then spend about three weeks at home to recuperate. I'll make a nice, neat, low incision that will hardly be noticeable. You'll never have to worry about menstruation or cancer of the cervix or uterus again. You will have a foolproof birth-control method, so your husband won't have to get a vasectomy."

One month later, Sally died on the operating table. Every year, over two thousand women die from hysterectomy surgery.[1] Hysterectomy is a major surgical procedure, and any major surgery carries with it the risk of death from the surgery itself, from anesthesia, or from postoperative complications. Hysterectomy patients also risk emotional problems, especially when complications occur during convalescence. These patients have to recover from surgical problems and from the physical and mental problems associated with estrogen loss and castration.

Nevertheless, hysterectomy is one of the most popular

surgical procedures done in the United States: 800,000 each year. At a cost of approximately $1,000 each, hysterectomies account for nearly $800 million in surgical fees per year. More than half of American women will undergo this sugery by the time they are 65 years old.[2] Thirty percent (240,000 women) will have nonfatal complications, ranging from fever and wound infections to bladder and bowel perforations. Another 15 percent (120,000 women) will require transfusions and run a significant risk of contracting hepatitis.[3]

Women who have hysterectomies are five times as likely to have severe depression that requires psychiatric care as women who do not have any surgery, and they are twice as likely to need psychiatric care as women who have had other types of abdominal surgery. More than half of the women under 40 who have hysterectomies will suffer severe postoperative depression.[4]

Despite these facts, some physicians think that we are not doing enough hysterectomies; they argue that every woman should have one to prevent cancer. Oddly enough, not one male physician I know advocates preventive prostatectomies (removal of the prostate gland) for men, although according to the American Cancer Society, just about the same number of deaths are caused annually by prostate cancer in men and uterine cancer in women. And the threat to women is not as great, since cancer of the cervix or uterus is so much easier to detect early than cancer of the prostate. Nevertheless, while urologists never do prophylactic prostate surgery, gynecologists routinely recommend prophylactic hysterectomy for women. Why do women merit such undue concern? Are we simply victims of a sexist system?

About ten years ago, a meeting of the American College of Obstetrics and Gynecology debated whether hysterectomies performed solely for birth control (sterilization) were justified. At the conclusion of the debate, the gynecologists in the audience voted by applauding. According to the audiometer that measured the loudness of the hand clapping, the proponents of hysterectomy for sterilization won.[5] There is no doubt in my mind that the vote would have gone the other way, overwhelmingly, if they had been debating the justification of castrating males for sterilization. Today, in spite of the women's rights movement, the ERA, and a generation of consciousness raising, more and more women every year enter operating rooms in this country to have hysterectomies and also be castrated (most people don't know that "castration" mean "removal of the testicles *or* ovaries").

Meanwhile, organized medicine continues to debate whether all these hysterectomies are necessary; but the debate cannot be resolved because medical men cannot even agree on the criteria for a necessary hysterectomy. Many studies have reviewed the medical records of women who have had hysterectomies. The pro-hysterectomy studies conclude, of course, that almost all the hysterectomies performed are necessary. The anti-hysterectomy studies conclude that as many as 40 percent of hysterectomies reviewed were unnecessary.[6] Gynecologists are still reacting to these studies, and many are doing their own.

There are some indications that nearly everyone would agree call for hysterectomy. These are:

cancer of the uterus, ovaries, or vagina
obstetrical hemorrhage where hysterectomy is necessary to save the woman's life
uterine prolapse, the medical term for a uterus that has dropped, sometimes to the point where the cervix is protruding outside the vagina (This results from childbirth and is caused by loss of muscular support for the uterus due to stretching or tearing. The uterus itself in this case may be quite normal.)
large fibroids causing symptoms of pressure or bleeding that cannot be medically controlled
cancers or infections of nearby tissues which have spread to involve the uterus

Beyond these criteria, there is much less agreement on exactly what conditions require hysterectomy. In one recent study, for example, a doctor reviewed 3,484 hysterectomy charts (that included three deaths) and reported that 12 percent of the surgeries had diagnoses of chronic cervicitis (inflammation of the cervix due to infection), noncancerous polyps (overgrowth of tissue), or nothing at all. Uterine prolapse or pelvic relaxation accounted for another 20 percent. Seventy percent of the hysterectomies followed diagnoses of cancer and "other clearly identified uterine pathology."[7] This statement suggests that in 70 percent of the cases, hysterectomy is winning an overwhelming victory over cancer, but the implication is terribly misleading. In reality, only 6 percent of these women had cancer. The other 64 percent had fibroids (benign tumors consisting mainly of fibrous tissue) or adenomyomas (benign tumors containing muscle and glandular tissue); and although fibroids are "clearly defined pathology," they usually do not constitute a justifiable reason for hysterectomy.

The doctor concludes that "This review, undertaken to see if unnecessary hysterectomy dominates the surgical scene, shows that the procedure is justified and not a rip-off of the public."[8] Yet when one adds to the 12 percent that he conceded were unnecessary the 64 percent done to remove fibroids and adenomyomas, it is hard to accept his conclusion.

Another recent study was made at a hospital associated with Wayne State University by Doctors Hassan Amirikia and T. N. Evans. Dr. Evans concluded that "the large number who were operated on for bleeding without demonstrated [abnormalities] is really no longer acceptable. Very, very few patients should ever have a hysterectomy just because of bleeding."[9] And both doctors noted that the "risks do not seem to justify utilizing this operation for the sole purpose of sterilization, in preference to simpler and safer procedures." Among the 6,435 hysterectomy patients studied by Amirikia and Evans, 17 died and 1,235 (more than 1 in 6) suffered complications; yet despite the facts of their own study, the doctors concluded: "Probably few operations will ever contribute as much to improving the quality of life of women as do indicated hysterectomies."[10] Apparently the researchers had made up their minds in advance and could not be swayed by data that failed to match their pre-conceptions.

Most hysterectomies are "elective"—that is, scheduled ahead of time and done for non–life-threatening purposes. Where a particular physician stands on the criteria for elective procedures depends on who trained him, peer pressure, and, in some measure, how much he wants to do the surgery. (Most surgeons feel that surgery they are trained to perform, and which they do very well, is good for the patient, and so they do not hesitate to recommend it.) Some physicians will only recommend an elective hysterectomy for conservative indications such as a fibroid uterus which is at least twelve to fourteen weeks in size (the size it would be at three to three and a half months of pregnancy) or pelvic relaxation as a result of childbirth, with resultant problems such as urinary leakage and difficult bowel evacuation. (In this latter situation, hysterectomy is a necessary adjunct to the extensive surgery necessary to repair these bothersome problems.) Other physicians will recommend the operation for such marginal reasons as sterilization, uterine polyps, menstrual pain, and cervical infections. Some physicans also recommend hysterectomy for cancer prevention. (If you do not have a uterus, you can never get uterine cancer.) The major justification for elective hysterectomy is that it will make life better for the woman, either on a purely physical basis or by giving her mental assurance that her problems are over.

Obviously, if a woman is in distress and is bleeding or she has other major, life-threatening symptoms, the decision for surgery is easy to make. However, when a woman who has no serious symptoms is told that she needs a hyster-ectomy, for whatever reason, the decision is more difficult. She is understandably ambivalent. She fears cancer, she fears the surgery, and she also fears that if she postpones surgery, her minor problems might grow into big, dangerous ones. She also fears the disapproval of her doctor. Unfortunately, no one can guarantee that everything will be all right if she chooses to wait. The surgeon implies, however, that if she has the hysterectomy now, at least she won't have to worry anymore.

And so it is easy to "sell" a hysterectomy to a woman who does not need one. The suggestion that a hysterectomy will solve your problems, provide life-long birth control, guarantee that you won't ever get cancer of the uterus or cervix, and rid you of the bother of painful menstruation can be very appealing. The sexism of the surgeon's recommendation becomes apparent when you consider that menstrual cramps, which have never been deemed significant enough to study and treat medically, are considered ample reason, in some cases, for elective hysterectomy. Menstrual pain, so long thought to be the invention of hysterical females, is transformed from a psychological problem to a significant gynecological problem requiring major surgery in the mind of the surgeon.

In my own fine teaching institution, the expression most often heard regarding hysterectomy is, "If there's doubt, take it out!" Men have become accustomed to ignoring or minimizing a woman's feelings for her uterus and ovaries; they simply don't know how women feel, and they don't bother to think about it. For the past fifteen years, I have eaten lunch with male colleagues who carry on lively discussions on hysterectomy procedures. They quip and smile and nod back and forth knowingly while enjoying their dull hospital fare. A few months ago, however, I had breakfast with eight male doctors at a country-club meeting of a medical society. The conversation suddenly swung to one of the men who was involved in the rather unusual sex-change surgery on men. The surgeon began explaining in detail how he made the incision and freed the testes prior to taking them out. At that point, one of the doctors at the table quietly put down his knife and fork, got up, and left, I was enjoying the excellent food—superb ham and eggs, freshly squeezed orange juice, hot rolls dripping with butter—and the usual sort of clinical conversation; but as the surgeon kept on talking about how he finally removed the testes and made an incision around the base of the penis, I noticed the doctor to my left fidgeting. The doctor to my right crossed his legs, quickly followed by two others who in their haste pulled the tablecloth this way and that. I began to realize that all was not well with my colleagues. Suddenly one of them, no longer able to take the conversation with his breakfast, snapped, "For Christ's sake, that's enough, Jerry, change the subject!"

I didn't say much during the conversation. I wasn't the least bit upset and hadn't even crossed my legs once. In retrospect, I know that if the conversation had been on hysterectomies that morning, my eight male colleagues would have enjoyed their breakfast. I know, too, that I can never have the empathy or innate feeling about male castration that a man feels. Male organs are just not a part of my own body reference.

Unlike the male gonads, woman's organs are hidden. When a woman has a hysterectomy, with or without the removal of her ovaries, she's not missing anything visible. At least on the surface, nothing seems to have changed. So, from a male perspective, a hysterectomy is no big deal. Why would any normal, sane woman who has finished having her family want a uterus anyway? And so it is not hard to understand why competent, conscientious physicians are positive that hysterectomy is a boon to womankind.

And to many women patients, more or less passively acquiescing to the male medical establishment, hysterectomy, initially at least, seems like a sensible procedure. They are sold by the argument that they will never again be bothered with menstruation, birth control, or unpredictable menopause.

I have yet to have a patient in my own private practice tell me that she wants a hysterectomy because she thinks she will be much happier without her uterus. It is possible that my patient population is not representative. I am a family doctor, not a surgeon. This probably influences the type of patient who comes to me. It certainly influences how I treat my patients. I chose medicine, rather than surgery, because I do not have a surgical personality. (Either you are a cutter or you are not. Either you love surgery or you avoid it like the plague. This decision is usually made early in medical school.) Being a noncutter and, therefore, not especially fond of bloody surgical procedures, I often influence my patients to bide their time, especially when it comes to elective surgery, whether it is a hysterectomy, a tonsillectomy, or back surgery.

Over the past fifteen years, I have referred only three women for hysterectomies. Two had cancer (one of the cervix and the other of the endometrium) and the third had a large fibroid-filled uterus that was causing her to become anemic. I am currently contemplating a fourth referral.

On the other hand, at least one of every three women in my practice has already had a hysterectomy before she becomes my patient; and of the hundreds of these women who have had previous hysterectomies, only three had them because of cancer. What, then, were the reasons that all these women underwent major surgery?

Almost all of these women had hysterectomies for fibroids, unusual bleeding, or "precancerous" conditions of the uterine lining. None of them, when pressed for additional data, really understood much of what went into the decision-making process that led to her hysterectomy. None knew the actual size of her uterus. None knew just how dangerous her "precancerous" condition was or if it could have been treated medically. None was aware that medical therapy might have gotten her through her bleeding problem long enough for menopause to ultimately solve the problem.

My practice has more than its share of lawyers, engineers, and other professional women. All of them had signed so called informed-consent forms for surgery. Yet none of these women was able to provide more than a vague general impression to explain why her hysterectomy had been done. They all were very *un*informed, in fact.

If my group of sophisticated, educated women don't know what made their surgery necessary, I can only assume that most women don't understand why they had to have surgery either.

Too many hysterectomies are routinely performed on women who have abnormal bleeding patterns, such as irregular or heavy menstrual flow, although these problems often are symptoms of hormonal imbalances that can be treated medically. Most of the time, the reason is an absence or shortage of progesterone, a female hormone produced in the ovary, and the "cure" is to supply more progesterone. Patient and physician may have to experiment to find the proper dosage and the best way to administer the hormone, but persistence usually brings positive results.

In one particularly stubborn case, after doing a complete workup to rule out cancer and other problems, I started a 41-year-old patient on progesterone tablets. Her heavy bleeding decreased a little but went on. After ten months, a D & C was done and a consultant gynecologist placed her on birth-control pills. After three months with little improvement, the gynecologist suggested a hysterectomy. The patient, however, did not want surgery, so I suggested that we try a progesterone-containing IUD, on the theory that its progesterone would act directly on her uterine lining and decrease her bleeding. Within a short time, her bleeding pattern became and has since remained normal.[11]

Another very common diagnosis that often leads to hysterectomy is fibroids (leiomyomas). A fibroid is a benign (noncancerous), solid growth within the muscular wall of the uterus, enclosed in a capsule which separates it from the uterine wall itself. Fibroids may be singular or multiple. They may be located in the middle of the uterine wall, or near the outside, or in the inner portion of the wall nearest the uterine cavity. If there are several small fibroids in the uterus, the uterus may retain its general contour but seem to be enlarged. On the other hand, if a growing fibroid is located on the outer portion of the wall and pokes out from the surface, the contour of the uterus feels irregular and bumpy to the doctor during the pelvic examination.

Fibroids usually feel firm because of the high proportion of hard, fibrous, gristlelike tissue they contain. Softer fibroids, usually found in the middle portion of the uterine wall or near the inner surface, contain more soft muscle fiber.

If you have fibroids that are located within the middle portion of the uterine wall or near the outer surface, more than likely you will have no symptoms. On the other hand, if your fibroids are located down near the inner surface or cavity of the uterus (submucous fibroids), you might have symptoms. Because of their position just beneath the uterine lining, these submucous fibroids are often associated with bleeding problems. The bleeding is often heavy and may occur in gushes during the normal menstrual period. These "flooding" episodes may leave you pale, anemic, and in need of both medical and surgical attention. Fortunately, submucous fibroids are rare, while fibroids in other positions are common.

Fibroids, even submucous fibroids, do not cause abnormal bleeding *patterns,* such as bleeding between menses or changes in the interval between menses. Bleeding-pattern problems are due to hormonal imbalances or, on rare occasions, to uterine cancer, and require investigation.

The diagnosis of uterine fibroids is usually made by physical examination during the annual or semiannual checkup. Most women are surprised to hear that they have fibroids, because they have no symptoms. Women with very large fibroids, however, may experience abdominal fullness or feel a mass arising in the lower abdomen. It is essential that you see your doctor if you have any such feelings or symptoms. Symptoms such as these may also be associated with other tumors that are dangerous, and an examination is imperative. (Of course, abdominal enlargement and firm growth in the lower abdomen is also associated with pregnancy ... musn't forget that possibility!)

It is important to know the size of your uterus and fibroids. Without such knowledge, it is impossible to participate intelligently in decisions such as whether to have surgery. For

example, suppose that during your examination in the doctor's office, you are told that your uterus contains fibroids
and is enlarged to the size of a three-month pregnancy.
If you know that your uterus has been that size for the
past four years, you will not be alarmed. On the other hand,
if your uterus was normal size just six months ago, this
is a significant finding, because fibroids that enlarge rapidly
may become cancerous. Only 0.5 percent of fibroids become
malignant[12] (called leiomyosarcomas), so the chances are
99.5 percent that your fibroids will be benign; but unless
you keep track of the size and condition of your uterus,
you won't be able to evaluate changes. Therefore, don't
settle for a doctor's knowing "ummm" as he examines you.
Speak up and ask him to describe what he feels. (This information can also be very useful to a doctor who is seeing
you for the first time. If you can tell him what previous
findings have been, he can more accurately evaluate your
uterine potential for future problems.)

Uterine fibroids usually do not require surgery unless they
cause symptoms. I am convinced by the available evidence
that unless there is a bona-fide reason to remove your uterus
immediately, you are well advised to forgo surgery and continue having regular checkups. If you have fibroids and the
size of your uterus is less than that of a three-and-a-half-
month pregnancy (twelve- to fourteen-weeks' size), and you
have no symptoms and no recent rapid increase in the size
of your fibroids, watch and wait. Fibroids are very common
and are found in nearly one-third of women approaching
menopause. They are rarely found in very young women
and seldom increase in size after menopause. In fact, fibroids
and the uterus tend to decrease in size with the onset of
menopause. If symptoms develop, surgery can always be
done; but if you can hold surgery off until menopause begins,
you probably can avoid it altogether.

Sometimes it's hard to watch and wait. You're not quite
sure what's going to happen during the next few months.
You have become a participant in the decision-making process and may feel burdened by sharing the responsibility.

You also must face going to your doctor's office full of anxiety and wondering if changes have occurred that will push your fate one way or another. Even worse, if you sought a second opinion, one surgeon probably counseled you to watch and wait while the other recommended that you get it over with now. As I write this, I have a patient who is going through this dilemma, but we (she and I) have decided to watch and wait. She has no desire for surgery. More important, she has no symptoms, and her uterine lining is normal. Although her uterus is about the size of a fourteen-week pregnancy and no one would ever raise an eyebrow if she had surgery, we will wait and keep our fingers crossed that there will be no further increase in the size of her fibroids or symptoms, and that her menopause begins soon. When that happens, shrinkage both in uterine size and fibroid size will occur. Meanwhile, surgery is always available, but will be used only as a last resort. It may be difficult to be in her position, but there are no surgical deaths to complicate waiting and seeing.

If you have fibroids causing such problems that surgery is indicated, but you want to have more children, it is possible, through a surgical procedure called myomectomy, to remove just the fibroids and leave the uterus intact. If you have this surgery, there is a 10 percent chance that new fibroids will appear. There is a slightly higher death rate for this procedure than for hysterectomy.[13] And when you become pregnant, the delivery most likely will be by cesarean section.

Most hysterectomies are preceded by an office endometrial biopsy or a D & C, a gyncological procedure for removing tissue from the lining of the uterus for biopsy. Some women are told after this procedure that they have "premalignant" or "precancerous" disease, and they naturally fear that although they do not have cancer yet, they surely will have it soon.

Actually, the term "premalignant disease" is a misnomer for many diagnoses. Furthermore, the actual chances that any particular "premalignant condition" will ever become cancerous are rarely discussed. And so many women, convinced that they are avoiding cancer, consent to hysterectomy.

The following section is for the woman who has been told that she has premalignant disease. It contains current statistics on the cancer potential of various precancerous diagnoses and other information to help her evaluate her options. This section contains a lot of technical names and terms, so if you have no such diagnosis to worry about, you may choose to go on without reading about premalignant disease.

"PRECANCEROUS" CONDITIONS
(Are they just another excuse for hysterectomy?)

The endometrium (the lining of the uterus) is shed each month during menses. This soft tissue and the blood it contains form most of the bloody discharge of the menstrual period. Only the innermost or basal layer of the endometrium does not slough off each month. It remains and forms the base for the growth of the new lining each month.

That growth of the endometrium is interrupted each month by menstruation. With the menses, the old cells are washed out and replaced by fresh new ones as the uterine lining rebuilds itself.

Estrogen, a female hormone secreted by the ovaries, stimulates the activities that occur in the first half of the monthly cycle, when the cells of the uterine lining increase in number and glands begin to grow. This is known as the proliferative phase of the monthly cycle. Ovulation occurs at mid-month (approximately) and triggers the second phase of the cycle. Ovulation cues the ovaries to secrete a second female hormone, progesterone, and this phase of the cycle continues under the control of both estrogen and progesterone. The uterine lining prepares for the possible implantation of a fertilized egg; glands increase in number and secrete sugar-containing substances to nourish the implanting egg. Since this part of the cycle, known as the secretory phase, is triggered by ovulation, it occurs only when ovulation has taken place.

In normal menstruating women, the mechanism for ovulation may not function perfectly each month. Sometimes a "normal" woman (especially the woman approaching menopause) may not produce an egg for one to four months out of each and every year. Sometimes there is a lighter or heavier menstrual flow at the end of these months; at other times, there is no flow and the woman "misses" a period. Should there be two or three consecutive months without menstruation, the endometrium will continue to grow uninterrupted. Cells and glands that would have been sloughed off at menstruation accumulate. This overabundance of cells is called hyperplasia. To a pathologist examining such endometrial tissue under the microscope, the cells look a little crowded, and the pathologist will call the resultant overcrowding *slight* hyperplasia. In the woman with four or more consecutive anovulatory cycles (cycles in which no egg is produced) he will call the condition hyperplasia.[14]

The patient with endometrial hyperplasia may be told that she has a premalignant disease; and she may, as a result, have a hysterectomy. But hyperplasia is only one of the changes in the endometrium that are inaccurately called premalignant.

Pathologists have a scoring scale to describe a progression of conditions from the most normal endometrium—least likely to be associated with endometrial cancer—to the most abnormal—most likely to be associated with the future onset of endometrial cancer. The scale is set up like a teeter-totter. At one end is the normal secretory endometrium, and at the opposite end is endometrial cancer. Next to secretory endometrium is proliferative endometrium—the normal endometrium seen during the first part of the cycle, when no progesterone is present; next, hyperplasia; next, cystic hyperplasia; closer to the center is adenomatous hy-

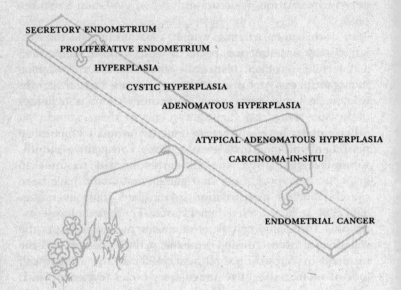

perplasia; and just across the fulcrum and somewhat on the far, or cancer, side of the teeter-totter is atypical adenomatous hyperplasia. Don't give up on the names: it's easy to catch onto the pathological jargon. The teeter-totter concept is the important part, because it gives you some idea of the potential malignancy of your diagnosed condition. Let's look at each condition in turn, beginning with the least threatening: hyperplasia.

In *hyperplasia,* it's the failure to ovulate that creates the problem, because ovulation failure is coupled with failure of the ovary to secrete progesterone. You need progesterone to maintain a normal endometrium. So if you haven't ovulated for a few months, that is no reason to throw in the towel and have a hysterectomy. Progesterone, in the form of tablets or a monthly injection, will easily change your endometrium back to its normal condition. The dosage of progesterone is important, because it must be sufficient to make up for all the progesterone that you lack each month. I have had success with 100 milligrams of progesterone in oil as a monthly injection, or 100 milligrams of Provera per month. Norlutate and other progesterones are fine, too. Your own doctor will probably have his favorite. Almost all women with hyperplasia can be treated with progesterone or by a D & C, which removes the overgrown population of cells; or both.

Hyperplasia is rarely "premalignant." Only 1 to 2 percent of women who get endometrial cancer have had simple hyperplasia eight to twelve years earlier.[15] That means that 98 to 99 percent of women with endometrial hyperplasia will *not* develop uterine cancer. However, there are some very rare situations where the diagnosis of hyperplasia may carry the threat of cancer. A woman who has a family history of endometrial cancer or gastrointestinal cancer is at risk with hyperplasia; but she has also had some years to think and to do something about her condition. That something need not be hysterectomy, and certainly should not be an overhasty one.

Cystic hyperplasia is a somewhat more intense buildup of cells in the endometrium caused by the same process as hyperplasia. Probably some six months of uninterrupted growth is necessary for cystic hyperplasia to develop.[16] Under the microscope, each cell is normal in appearance, although there are far too many of them; but the secretory glands of the endometrium appear to be fat, rounded, and lined by more crowded cells.

This condition can be treated medically by progesterone or removed by a D & C, and in about two-thirds of cases, it will not recur. If it does come back, it can be removed again by a D & C. Cystic hyperplasia goes on to become endometrial cancer some eight to ten years later in 0.4 percent of patients.[17] Thus 99.6 percent of women with cystic hyperplasia will not develop endometrial cancer; and as in simple hyperplasia, there is a long time span between this problem and the development of cancer. So take your time; consider that 99.4 percent is a pretty solid edge to have, and relax. Don't forget, however, to take your progesterone and have regular checkups.

Adenomatous hyperplasia brings us a little closer to the middle of the teeter-totter. For me, adenomatous hyperplasia sits squarely on the side of the board with the normals, but some would debate this premise. In this condition, the overgrowth of cells (all of which are normal in appearance) has reached a very crowded state. The rounded glands now have changed and show infoldings and outfoldings at their borders. With adenomatous hyperplasia, the percentage of women who go on to develop cancer increases dramatically. Up to 15 percent of women with this condition will get endometrial cancer. And the cancer usually will develop only three to five years after adenomatous hyperplasia is found by D & C.[18]

Most of my patients who have had hysterectomies (prior to becoming my patients) for "precancerous" changes of the uterine lining have had that surgery because they had adenomatous hyperplasia. I doubt that all of these hysterectomies were necessary. Certainly there are other options.

In the first place, 85 percent of women with adenomatous hyperplasia will not develop cancer of the uterus. And adenomatous hyperplasia, like simpler hyperplastic conditions, can be treated medically by progesterone. At the very least, a trial of progesterone will not harm the patient and will most likely result in a normal uterine lining within a few months. The abnormal lining also can be removed by D & C. Two-thirds of women with adenomatous hyperplasia will not regrow a hyperplastic uterine lining after one D & C, and another 20 percent will be "cured" by a second D & C. In one study of 500 D & Cs, the remaining 12 percent of women whose hyperplastic condition recurred either had a third D & C or a hysterectomy, or both, and no cancer was present.[19] Having a hospital D & C may seem like a lot of bother, but believe me, even repeated D & Cs are less bothersome than a single hysterectomy. (Even easier is the newly developed procedure of aspiration-suction biopsy in your doctor's office.*) I have treated adenomatous hyperplasia patients with progesterone—a 10-milligram tablet for ten days each month—followed by office aspirations some four to six months later. (All of them had normal-size uteri and no suspicious findings on their pelvic examinations.) The uterine linings of all of them returned to normal.

Many women who have hyperplasias are approaching menopause, when the ovary loses its ability to produce an egg and trigger progesterone secretion. If these women can be held over for several months, most of them will become menopausal, which usually solves the problem. The menopausal uterine lining rarely has the capability to regrow after a D & C. Therefore, a D & C which interrupts the process should be enough to "cure" the patient.

Should adenomatous hyperplasia occur in a young woman, it is more aggressive and more prone to develop into cancer. This phenomenon is rare—only 4 percent of endometrial cancer occurs in women under 40 years of age—and it also tends to occur in women with family histories of cancer.[20] It is also seen in women who never or almost never ovulate because of some chromosomal abnormality or long-lasting problem, such as Stein-Leventhal syndrome. Women in these groups bear special watching and should have more aggressive care.

Atypical adenomatous hyperplasia is a step much closer to the development of cancer in the uterine lining. In this condition, for the first time, the individual cells of the endometrium begin to look unnatural. Some of them are too dark, while others seem to be piled in a jumbled arrangement without any apparent pattern. Their appearance is no longer neat and clean but disordered. Usually lots of white blood cells are mixed through the tissue, as if they were trying to clean up some of the mess.

Studies have found that in many cases, this condition was

*See intrauterine aspiration (pages 253–55).

diagnosed one to three years before cancer was diagnosed.
Still, only 15 percent of the women with endometrial atypical
adenomatous hyperplasia are believed to progress to cancer.[21] Here, too, 85 percent of women with this condition
do not regrow the abnormal uterine lining after a D & C
and do not develop cancer.

If a patient came into my office and told me (or I learned
after receiving her pathology report from the hospital) that
she had had a hysterectomy because she had atypical adenomatous hyperplasia, I would think that she had been given
reasonable treatment. But she might instead have had a carefully monitored trial on progesterone and thereby have
avoided surgery (other than periodic office aspirations or
hospital D & Cs, which are minor).

The condition called *carcinoma-in-situ* involves more than
a simple change in the endometrium. It is cancer of the
uterine lining that has not invaded the muscular wall of
the uterus. It is an uncommon cancer that seems to occur
at the average age of 50. It is thought that carcinoma-in-
situ is irreversibly programmed to progress, invading the
surrounding tissue, unless it is destroyed, removed, or al-
tered by hormonal therapy. Some cases have been reversed
by progesterone therapy. The usual treatment, however, is
hysterectomy. As frightening as it sounds, endometrial carcinoma-in-situ may take from one to ten years to become
an invasive cancer.[22] Thus it is still not a surgical emergency,
and you may want to take your time to double-check the
diagnosis.

These, then, aside from invasive uterine cancer, are the
various diagnoses you might be given after an endometrial
biopsy or a D & C. It is important that you see your pathology
sheet and read the two or three words that follow the diagnosis. Only in that way can you know for sure your exact
diagnosis and just what the "premalignant changes" are.
Then you can compare your diagnosis with the material presented here and decide for yourself just how urgent your

"indicated hysterectomy" is. If your diagnosis is adenomatous hyperplasia, atypical adenomatous hyperplasia, or carcinoma-in-situ, you should have your slides reviewed by a pathologist who has special expertise in uterine problems. Some pathologists are not as well trained in endometrial abnormalities as others, although for the diagnosis of plain hyperplasia or cystic hyperplasia, your everyday pathologist should be expert enough.

As sometimes happens, pathologists who are not experts on the endometrium may look at a slide, decide that it "looks bad," and without ever actually coming to a diagnosis, advise the surgeon that the uterus probably should come out. He and the surgeon both feel that it is better to err on this side rather than to leave some "bad-looking" lining and risk getting sued later if the patient develops cancer.

You should not have a hysterectomy just because your endometrium "looks bad." Get a specific diagnosis, preferably from a pathologist experienced in uterine problems, before you even consider hysterectomy. Furthermore, neither plain hyperplasia nor cystic hyperplasia should ever be the only basis for your decision for hysterectomy, unless, of course, there are other associated problems that are not being considered here.

And now you know just about as much uterine pathology as most nonpathologist doctors. I did not add that statement to be funny. I added that statement because it is sad and true.

OVARIES: IN OR OUT?

If you do have a hysterectomy, you will face the question: should the ovaries be removed when your hysterectomy is done? This is a question that you and your doctor should carefully consider. If you are postmenopausal, there is usually little choice. Your ovaries are not functioning (or produce hormones only at low levels) and they are a potential site of ovarian cancer and other problems and should be removed. However, some doctors always automatically remove

ovaries if the patient is over 50 years of age. Others use
45 as their cut-out age, while still others are beginning to
take out ovaries at age 40. Anytime a doctor tells you that
he automatically removes anything at any given age, worry!
Each patient should be evaluated individually.

Premenopausal women should not consider removal of
the ovaries unless there is a family history of ovarian or
breast cancer. In these cases, or if upon opening the abdomen, the ovaries are seen to be diseased or nonfunctional
and shriveled, they should be removed. If you are premenopausal, the removal of your ovaries will mean that you
may experience the sudden onset of menopausal symptoms,
including hot flashes and night sweats. Oral estrogen-replacement therapy may relieve these problems. But simply
replacing estrogen can't fulfill the many other functions of
the ovaries: their role in metabolism, in regulating other
endocrine organs, in protecting against development of osteoporosis, and perhaps cardiovascular disease. We know
the ovaries produce multiple hormones. But we still don't
know the full effects on the body of the ovaries—or the
loss of the ovaries.

The January 1981 issue of the *American Journal of Obstetrics
and Gynecology* reported that surgical removal of both ovaries
in young women is associated with an increase in myocardial
infarction (heart attack). Women who have only one ovary
removed, however, have only a slight increase in risk. The
younger the woman, the greater the risk. For example, the
removal of both ovaries from women under 35 years of
age increases the risk of myocardial infarction seven times
that over normal. As 25 percent of women undergoing hysterectomy have both ovaries removed, it would follow that
we will see an increasing number of heart attacks among
women who are subjected to this practice.

The doctors who advocate the removal of the ovaries do
so because they hope to prevent the later development of
ovarian cancer. Studies have shown, however, that when the
uterus alone is removed and the ovaries are left in place,

the incidence of cancer is no higher in the residual ovaries than it would be if the woman had not had her uterus removed. In other words, ovarian cancer may occur in the residual ovaries, but not at a rate greater than normal.

Leaving the ovaries means that the woman must return to her physician for simple pelvic checkups every six months to make sure that the ovaries remain normal-size. Luckily, ovarian problems are easier to detect after a hysterectomy, because the bulky uterus is no longer in the physician's way during the examination, and any question as to the size or consistency of the ovaries can be checked by sonogram, a painless examination using sound waves (see pages 257–58). The premenopausal woman who loses her uterus, then, is better off keeping her semiannual appointments— and her ovaries.

There is another reason—besides the risk of serious complications or even death from unnecessary surgery—that hysterectomy should not be taken lightly. Depression is a common aftermath. It usually occurs within three to six months after surgery and can be severe enough to require institutionalization.

Our society and culture have conditioned women to think of our inherent worth in terms of our sexuality, especially as it relates to childbearing ability, either actual or potential. The removal of the uterus (the focus of childbearing) may lead us to feel incomplete, neutered, unattractive, and no longer able to give or receive sexual pleasure. The woman who loses her uterus may feel castrated. The woman who loses her ovaries as well has, in fact, been castrated.

The woman who has clear indications for the surgery— such as uterine cancer—rarely suffers from posthysterectomy depression because she has no ambivalence either before or after the surgery. Furthermore, she has no feelings of guilt or recrimination over a perhaps too hasty consent to surgery, since her life was at stake. Those women who undergo elective hysterectomies, on the other hand, run a great risk of depression. Even though a woman may accept the "need" for the surgery on an intellectual level, she has unresolved emotional stress. Like the victim of radical mastectomy, she may turn the rage she feels toward her surgeon inward against herself (depression).

Even though depression is a fairly predictable result of hysterectomy, it can be mitigated if the patient has proper support mechanisms. The physician is never adequate to this task, even if he is doing everything humanly possible. The two people who will have the greatest impact on how a patient adjusts to her hysterectomy are her mother and her husband.

Mother has already influenced many of the attitudes that we have concerning our self-image and sexuality. The presence of a mother during convalescence can be a potent factor, either enhancing or retarding psychological convalescence.

Clearly if your mother weeps and moans over the fact that you can no longer bear children, commiserates with you because you will no longer be desirable to your husband, and fills your head with all sorts of old-fashioned tales ("Aunt Sophie was never the same after her hysterectomy"), she should not be near you during your convalescence. On the other hand, if she is supportive, let her help you at this time; mothers usually are a great comfort to have near.

As for your husband, psychologist Martha N. Gizynski describes the typical behavior patterns of husbands:

> The supportive husband reassures his wife that she is still attractive to him, that he sees her as the same important person as before, and that their relationship is in no way altered. He is appropriately supportive of her dependency needs during her convalescence.
>
> The absent husband does not come for a preoperative consultation and does not show up at the hospital on the day of the surgery, but sends the patient's mother.
>
> The dependent husband has an overriding need to be taken care of himself, and is not capable of meeting the ordinary dependency needs of his wife, much less the escalated needs of a convalescing and emotionally shaken woman.

The guilty husband has neglected his wife in the past, for his career or for other women. Now that he is faced with the possibility that she will be seriously ill or will die, he overreacts and devotes himself day and night to anticipating her every need and wish. This makes his wife very uneasy, and she senses that she is going to have to die to make it all worthwhile.

The anxious husband may not be aware of it, but at some level he has identified with his wife and translated her surgery into an analogous procedure on himself. He sees her as castrated, and finds it threatening to live closely with a maimed person. He is not very supportive because he is trying to avoid facing the whole situation.

The jealous husband feels like an outsider. His wife is loyal and devoted to her physician who she quotes as gospel. She is somewhat less admiring of her husband. Understandably, he feels unloved and hurt.[23]

Your husband or lover may not intuitively realize how much you need his support; don't hesitate to ask for his help, and turn also to other family members or friends. Arrange to have a good friend spend time with you as you recuperate. Don't try to go it alone.

Hysterectomy may also cause problems with your sex life. Some women find that orgasm "feels different." The uterus, like the vagina, contracts during orgasm, so the loss of uterine sensation may contribute to sexual dissatisfaction. Other women complain of vaginal shortening or lessening of the vagina's ability to expand and contract during intercourse. These problems usually result from poor surgical technique, very extensive surgery, or loss of ovarian estrogen.

Lack of sexual desire is more likely to become a problem when the ovaries are removed during surgery, because the ovaries are a major source not only of female hormone, but also of male hormone thought to be especially important for your sex drive. Even estrogen replacement cannot correct that problem. The husband's sexual potential also may suffer. If a woman undergoes a hysterectomy for cancer, for example, the husband may feel that he might catch the cancer, or that he is the one who gave it to her. Such fears often lead to impotence. (On the other hand, the woman's sex life may improve, especially when pain or heavy bleeding or the possibility of pregnancy are no longer worries.)

Because your surgery affects both you and your husband, you both should be present for presurgical counseling. This becomes exceedingly important in those cases in which hysterectomy might pose a serious threat to the wife's sexual identity, either in the mind of the husband or wife. Alternatives to surgery should be discussed if there is evidence that marital instability will result from the impending surgery. A thorough understanding of the possible problems and possible negative feelings prior to surgery can help prevent some of the psychologically negative aftermath.

Finally, you yourself will be responsible for avoiding depression. You must weigh all the factors that are involved before agreeing to elective hysterectomy. You should have help from your physician, a second opinion from another physician, and a frank and honest discussion of the surgery with your family, husband, or lover.

In the final analysis, the decision for an elective hysterectomy must be made by the woman. If she succumbs to the seduction of a hysterectomy as a "cure-all," she will undoubtedly be dissatisfied with the results of the surgery, if not immediately, then surely over time. Hysterectomy is major surgery. It's not a procedure to decide upon capriciously. If this responsibility terrifies you, then you will find yourself at the mercy of your surgeon. The only important factor, then, becomes whether you have picked a conservative or an aggressive surgeon.

As things stand now, the burden of decision usually does not lie with the patient. In fact, hysterectomy studies reveal one very significant fact: the most important single factor influencing whether or not a woman has a hysterectomy is geography—where she lives.

Hysterectomy rates vary greatly from country to country, from state to state, and even from hospital to hospital. The hysterectomy rate in the United States is over twice the rate in England and Wales. The hysterectomy rate in the state of Vermont is greater than in the neighboring state of Maine. And the rate in northern Maine is greater than in southern Maine.

Efforts to explain this phenomenon have established that there is a very definite correlation between the hysterectomy rate in a given region and the number of gynecologists and surgeons who practice there. Vermont has more gynecologists and surgeons than Maine, so Vermont women have more hysterectomies per capita than Maine women.[24]

But assuming that you are not willing to abdicate your responsibility to a geographical accident, listen carefully. Do not be seduced by the promise that you will be immune to cervical and uterine cancer. Remember that regular Pap smears will pick up abnormalities of the cervix long before cancer occurs. Uterine aspiration also will alert you to endometrial changes before they become serious. There is plenty of time for a hysterectomy.

Surgeons are too willing to suggest and perform hysterectomies. Remember that contraception, dysmenorrhea, simple fibroids, and even many endometrial changes are not adequate reasons for hysterectomy. If you have a D & C or aspiration, make sure that you see and understand your endometrial diagnosis. Take responsibility for your body, for you must be satisfied, at the very least, that a surgical assault on your body is absolutely necessary. Otherwise your irresponsibility may affect your entire future, physically and mentally.

If you have problems, you should know your alternatives. All too often, a lesser surgical procedure or medical therapy will be sufficient, yet women continue to be pressured into riskier surgery. But if we women finally realize the need to inform ourselves about what goes on in our bodies and take responsibility for the medical decisions that may have to be made about them, then we will be well on our way to stopping the unnecessary carnage.

CHAPTER 7

Your Gynecological Examination: More for Your Money

The old saying "What you don't know can't hurt you" certainly does not apply to women's health care. What you don't know about your own reproductive organs can hurt you very much indeed. For that reason, it's not only important to have a Pap smear and a pelvic examination as a matter of routine health care, but also to understand what other things your doctor is checking for and why.

THE PAP SMEAR AND CERVICAL CANCER

The Pap smear or Pap test created a new era in female cancer detection, and when used routinely, it has the potential for virtually doing away with deaths from cervical cancer. It takes its name from George Papanicolaou, who, in the 1940s, developed a method of collecting, examining, and interpreting changes in cells shed by the cervix. The cervix, like the skin and the inside of the mouth, sheds millions of old cells every day and replaces them with new ones. To collect cells for the Pap test, a speculum made of metal or plastic is inserted into the vagina to open it. Then, using a light source, the physician can see the cervix. Using a long cotton applicator (much like a queen-size Q-tip) and a tiny wooden spatula (Ayre's spatula), he collects a sample of cells by rubbing the Q-tip and spatula over the cervix. The process takes only a minute or so and usually is completely painless. The cells that have been collected are then spread on glass slides and sprayed with a liquid to "fix" them. The spraying preserves the cells so that the lab can stain and examine them by microscope.

Most labs group Pap-smear results into five categories, though some labs use more. A Pap smear may be reported as Class I, II, III, IV, or V. Class I is normal. Class II indicates the presence of some inflammation. Generally this is due to infection or, sometimes in older women, to lack of estrogen. Clearing up the infection or giving the patient some local or oral estrogen may be all that is necessary to get that Pap to revert back to a Class I. Class III signifies the presence of dysplasia, which means that abnormal changes are going on within the cells. Some of these changes may be due to infection. Degrees of dysplasia range from mild to severe. About one-third of the Class III Pap smears improve and revert back to Class I or Class II on their own. Another third remain the same, and the last third get worse and may develop into carcinoma-in-situ (cancer that is localized in early stages, and superficial).

A Class IV category usually means that carcinoma-in-situ is present or that there is good reason to suspect that cancer is present. Class V, the rarest of all, indicates cervical cancer that is no longer localized and superficial (like carcinoma-in-situ) but extends deeper, invading the cervical tissues.

But keep in mind that the transition from a normal to an abnormal Pap takes a long time. There is ample warning, and early changes can be dealt with easily. No one should *ever* die from cervical cancer. If you have regular checkups, you will never have to worry.

But keep in mind, also, that although the Pap test is 90 to 95 percent accurate in diagnosing cervical cancer, it is not infallible. False negatives and positives do occur for many reasons. If the slides are not sprayed immediately after the specimen cells are collected, distortions of the cells may occur, or the technician examining the slide may misinterpret it. Sometimes a cancerous area is so small that neither the swab nor the wooden spatula picks up cells from the area. Sometimes the lab simply makes a mistake because the technician is not well trained or is required to read too many slides per day. (Fifty cases, or 100 slides, is the maximum a technician should be required to read a day.) Because Pap smears are not 100 percent reliable, women should return for yearly screenings. Then even if an abnormality is missed one year, it will most likely be picked up the next year.

The American Cancer Society (ACS) recently approved new cancer-screening guidelines for asymptomatic women. They recommend that Paps be done every three years, instead of annually (after two consecutive yearly Class I Paps). They reason that such a policy change will save money and unburden limited medical services. They also feel that cervical cancer grows very slowly and that, if the early stages of cancer are present, they can be detected years before they progress on to invasive cancer.

Nevertheless, about 5 percent of all cervical cancers develop rapidly, and a woman with one of these would stand little chance of early detection on an every-three-year Pap schedule. If a Pap was misread, six years is a long interval and bad news would likely get worse over such a long time span.

The most serious problem that I foresee resulting from three-year Pap intervals is that more women will die from advanced uterine and ovarian cancer and there will be a somewhat lesser increase in advanced cases of cervical cancer. Women have become accustomed to the annual Pap. If the annual Pap is discouraged, women will probably also forgo annual gynecological checkups, and miss the annual pelvic examination that is the only edge against these diseases. Waiting three years can be the difference between life and death, especially for ovarian cancers. If the ACS issues new Pap guidelines, they must educate women that annual pelvic exams are still necessary.

Pap smears should begin with the onset of sexual activity rather than at a specific age. If you are 16 and have been sexually active, you should have a Pap. On the other hand, if you are 18 and have never had intercourse, a Pap could be done but is most likely unnecessary, unless you have a specific complaint. By 21, most of my patients have had their first Pap.

My patients then come in for a yearly Pap until they are 40. After 40, they are seen every six months, not so much for a Pap as for a pelvic examination to make sure that the uterus and ovaries are and remain normal. (This exam, which will be discussed later, becomes more and more important as you age, because of the increasing incidence of cancer with increasing age.) There is no upper age limit for having a Pap smear. Most women feel that routine visits to the doctor can stop when they become menopausal. Nothing could be further from the truth. The older you are, the greater your chances of getting cancer. The older you are, the more you should keep appointments. Paps and more especially pelvic exams should be continued at least until you are 65 plus.

There is one exception to this rule—hysterectomy. For patients who have had a hysterectomy for the more usual reasons (i.e., fibroids, prolapse), I do a Pap once every five years, but I do an annual or semiannual pelvic exam to check their ovaries if they have not been removed. However, if you have had a hysterectomy because of cervical cancer or uterine or ovarian cancer, there is a remote possibility that abnormal cells might still exist which could begin to grow in the upper portion of the vagina. In such cases, annual screening for cervical cancer should be continued.

Getting women to take advantage of the Pap smear has been a mighty effort that has paid off in the saving of thousands of lives. The test takes just a few painless minutes in the doctor's office and it has saved many women by detecting their cancers before they spread. The Pap has also brought peace of mind to those millions of women who have negative findings.

* * *

Complete peace of mind about cervical cancer will of course only come when we are able to know what causes it and how it can be prevented. Although there are various theories, cervical cancer is thought to be a sexually transmitted (venereal) disease. It is almost never found in virgins or nuns, and most often found in women who have had sexual relations at an early age or who have had multiple partners. One reason for the first cause seems to be that the cells of the transformation area of the cervix (where cervical cancer almost always begins) are especially active during adolescence and pregnancy. During this active period, the cells are especially susceptible to stimuli that can cause cell transformation.

There are several theories to explain the sexual connection to cervical cancer. One is simply that women are infected by the herpes virus when having intercourse. This virus and other infections have been implicated as causative agents for many years.

Another theory places the blame directly on male sperm. Dr. Albert Singer of Sheffield, England, has collaborated with Dr. Bevan Reid of Sidney, Australia, on a study which strongly suggests that certain men are more likely than others to transmit cervical cancer.[1] There is some background for this hypothesis. A higher incidence of cervical cancer is found in women who are married to men who have cancer of the penis.[2] Another researcher, Kessler, found that the incidence of cervical cancer in the second, or in a few cases in the third, wives of men whose first wives had developed cervical cancer was 3.5 times higher than it should have been.[3] However, wives of vasectomized men have an incidence of cervical cancer lower than would be expected, according to Drs. Swan and Brown of the Kaiser-Permanente Medical Center.

All these findings seem to point to the fact that the sperm itself may carry a substance capable of causing cervical cancer, perhaps not in all women, but in susceptible women. Drs. Singer and Reid think that different men produce different amounts of histone or protamine, two basic proteins, in their sperm. These same proteins are also found in herpes virus, but the amount carried in the sperm is much greater.

These proteins may trigger the cellular changes that lead to cancer. According to Singer and Reid, men who have the highest ratios of these proteins in their semen tend to come from the lowest socioeconomic groups.[4] They found a straight-line comparison in the English and Australian population when they compared sperm chemistry with job type.

Their observation is further backed up by statistics. The standard mortality rate from cervical cancer is higher among women whose husbands have menial jobs, lower among women whose husbands are professionals, teachers, and the like. Statistics for England and Wales were reviewed for the years 1959–63, and this finding was reported in an article that appeared in *Lancet,* one of the major English medical journals.

Analyzing this kind of data can be very confusing. Is there something organically unique in high-risk men, or is it that these men (in certain occupations and at certain socioeconomic levels) fool around more, and therefore contract diseases that cause their wives problems later in life? Dr. Singer has told me in conversation, however, that he believes some particular men may be "high risk." He cited a case in which a teenager who had severe dysplasia of the cervix swore that she had had relations with only one young man. When her boyfriend was brought in and a semen sample obtained, its analysis revealed a tremendously high amount of protamine/histone.

The thinking in medical circles has been that women who develop cervical cancer most likely have had three or more sex partners. That assumption may not be valid. Perhaps it is more important *who* the partners are, because it may be that just one partner with unusual semen characteristics can be dangerous to your health.

I remember some ten years ago when I took a course in pathology and cytology, the physician teaching the course pointed out a slide that showed a sperm embedded in a cell from the cervix. He said that this was a common occurrence in unprotected intercourse. All of us knew that the entry of one cell into another could lead to cellular changes that might result in cancer.

Until we have some definitive studies about the exact role of sperm and herpes in causing cervical cancer, about the best one can do is advise young women, who are in the highest risk group for this kind of cancer, to be especially wary. I tell my teenage patients that the risk of cervical cancer is one of the best reasons I can think of for saying no to their boyfriends. Five minutes of pleasure is not worth chancing years of problems. I try not to moralize, because that is the function of the clergy. However, there are hard, cold, scientific facts about the coital etiology of cervical cancer that young women should not ignore. I tell teenagers that if they must have intercourse, they should insist that the man use a condom; the girl should use foam in order to get some additional protection from herpes, and should be sure to get Pap smears regularly.

THE PELVIC EXAM

While the Pap smear is the first line of detection for cervical cancer, it is only part of the reason for going to the doctor for a gynecological checkup. Women often mistakenly think they are cancer-free just because they have had a normal Pap. Nothing could be further from the truth. It's quite possible for a woman to have a normal Pap smear and die in two or three months from cancer of the uterus or ovary. The Pap, by itself, is not sufficient to screen for all forms of female cancer. The other and equally important portion of your visit to your doctor is the pelvic examination, which is your first line of defense for the detection of ovarian and uterine cancer and should always be performed whenever a Pap is done.

The doctor performs the pelvic exam immediately after taking the Pap. Two gloved and jellied fingers are introduced into the vagina (one, if the opening is small). The physician then puts his other hand on the lower portion of your abdomen and tries to outline your uterus and ovaries between the fingers of the hand on your abdomen and the fingers in your vagina.

The pelvic examination determines whether there are any abnormalities in the size or shape of the uterus and ovaries. It can also identify any area that is especially tender. During the examination, patients often become apprehensive. Ovaries often are tender, and women naturally assume that pain or discomfort during their pelvic examination automatically means that something is wrong. But discomfort is quite normal when the ovary is palpated. Sometimes the best way to teach young doctors to find ovaries is to have them watch the patient's face. If they are applying pressure and the patient suddenly shows a facial twinge of discomfort, more than likely they have found the ovary.

One of my young residents came up with an analogy that I have passed on to my own patients as a graphic, easily comprehended explanation for their fleeting discomfort. As I was demonstrating the proper technique of doing a good pelvic examination, the patient on the table said, "That area is a little bit tender."

I said to her, "That's normal; ovaries are always a little bit sensitive."

At that point, my resident piped up, "Yeah, they're like testicles; they're tender if you push on them." I have since shared that story with many a patient, who instantly comprehended and could then help me by relaxing.

The last part of your pelvic examination is a rectovaginal examination. This is accomplished by the physician placing one finger into the rectum while leaving one finger in the vagina. This gives the doctor the opportunity to evaluate tissue between the vagina and the rectum and to feel for tumors that could be growing in the posterior portion of the pelvis. It also provides an opportunity to make sure that there are no tumors in the lower rectum.

The pelvic examination should not just be one-two-three, zip. Although it takes only a minute or so, it must be done painstakingly and methodically. Sometimes it may not be. I have, on occasion, found pathology in women whose previous doctors had told them that the pain was in their heads.

You can help your doctor perform a successful pelvic examination. If you go to the bathroom immediately before, that will reduce the size of the bladder, which sits in front of the uterus and can prevent the palpation of structures that lie beneath it. If you tend to be constipated, a small enema before your appointment will get rid of hard stools that may confuse a physician trying to feel the structures in the pelvis.

D & C (DILATATION AND CURETTAGE)

While the Pap test exists specifically to test for cervical cancer, it sometimes detects uterine or ovarian cancer as well. The uterine lining, like the cervix, constantly sheds cells, much as a tree drops its leaves. Some of these cells fall onto the cervix, where they can be picked up by the cotton-tipped applicator. Other cells fall into the upper back portion of the vagina, where they also can be collected. Consequently, the Pap smear is able to detect about 50 percent of the cases of uterine cancer; but such a rate of detection is too small to be reliable. Better methods of screening for uterine cancer have come into use.

Various ways of collecting sample cells from the uterine lining have been developed. One frequently used is the D & C: "dilatation and curettage." Dilatation means stretching the opening of the cervical canal, a procedure that is necessary to allow the spoon-shaped curette to pass into the uterine opening. The curette has a sharp cutting edge to scrape off tissue samples of the uterine lining.

Both processes—dilatating the cervix and curetting the uterine lining—are painful, so the operation is done in a hospital under anesthesia. It is the most common operation done in the United States. Usually the D & C is a diagnostic procedure used to gather tissue for analysis, but it often is therapeutic, because it can remove the excess growth of tissue that is causing the problem. It is commonly used, for example, to arrest hyperplasia of the uterine lining by simply removing the overgrown lining.

INTRAUTERINE ASPIRATION

In recent years, simpler methods of collecting tissue samples right in the doctor's office have been devised. They usually involve the introduction of a narrow, hollow plastic or metal tube through the cervical opening and into the uterine cavity. Once inserted, the device is moved back and forth within the uterine cavity. Sometimes a syringe provides suction to withdraw cells from the surface of the lining through the strawlike tube, but more often the hollow tube is attached to an electric suction pump that sucks (aspirates) cells from the uterine lining down the tube into a collecting trap. Since the endometrial lining of the uterus is loose and fragile, suction alone collects ample amounts of cells and even tiny pieces of tissue. An experienced physician can obtain tissue that is nearly comparable to the tissue obtained from an actual D & C. A fixative is added to the aspirated tissue to preserve it and it is then sent to a lab, where it is stained and examined microscopically. The tissue samples reveal any abnormalities in the cells as well as how they relate to one another—information that is invaluable in making a diagnosis.

The office procedure of aspiration has many advantages that may make it preferable to a D & C. It costs less. It does not involve hospitalization or the risks of side effects of anesthesia. Patients usually feel some cramping at the time of the procedure, but the cramps stop as soon as the aspiration is over.

There are specific instances, however, where nothing less than a D & C will do. For instance, the cervical canal has to be open wide enough to admit the suction probe. Sometimes it is not possible to perform an aspiration in the office because the opening into the uterine cavity is closed too tightly, as in postmenopausal women whose menstruation stopped several months or years before. If polyps or other pathology is suspected, a hospital D & C may then, too, be the best procedure; although aspiration may diagnose the problem, it cannot remove the polyps as a D & C would.

More women should know about and take advantage of these newly available tests. With them, the reasons for intermenstrual spotting, prolonged menses, or heavy bleeding are easily discovered. Should there be anything terribly wrong, it will be diagnosed as soon as if a more extensive D & C had been performed.

Whenever I perform an aspiration on a patient, I tell her exactly what I am doing, from the moment I clean the area until I am finished. Once people know what is going on, they are less apprehensive. I ask patients to tell me if they are having any pain, and when they do, I stop immediately. The pain quickly subsides, the patient takes another deep breath, and we can continue. The patient must be in control of the situation.

Sometimes I have to check on a too-quiet patient. If I hear nothing from her, I stop after twenty seconds or so and look at her face. Since facial expressions tell the most, I usually can tell whether to continue or stop for a short pause. Some patients experience very little discomfort and wonder why I keep worrying about how they are feeling. Other patients give me very curt instructions:

"Get it over and let me get out of here!"

In any case, I pass the small, hollow, open-ended tube over the entire surface of the uterine lining, carefully going over the front, back, and side walls. I try not to miss any areas in my housecleaning attempt. I rattle off where I am, how much more I have to do, and my office nurse, Liz, offers a hand for my patient to hold onto if necessary.

Some women whose conditions have had to be constantly followed up because of pathology have had repeated aspirations. Nobody likes it, but the alternative is worse. In fact, gynecological examinations are universally disliked by most women. I could almost paint their words on the ceiling.

"I hate this most of all ... and going to the dentist is a close second."

OVARIAN CANCER

The ovary also sloughs cells, some of which pass down the fallopian tubes into the uterus and eventually wind up on the cervix or in the vagina. These cells may sometimes be spotted on a Pap smear, but because the path they have to travel to the cervix is so long and involved, they rarely are present. The Pap smear only diagnoses about 8 percent of the cases of ovarian cancer.

Ovarian cancer is a killer disease. The death rate is high because it is rarely diagnosed early. Of all pelvic malignancies, it is currently the leading cause of death.[5] Uterine and cervical cancer are easy to diagnose because we have good screening methods available, but none exists for ovarian cancer.

The disease occurs mostly among 40- to 60-year-old women, although a substantial amount (20 percent) occurs in women over the age of 60. If the lives of women with ovarian cancer are to saved, pelvic examinations must be carefully performed. I recently found ovarian tumors in three women who had come to me from "good" gynecologists. Ovaries are very difficult to palpate, and that is why a real effort must be made each and every time a doctor performs a pelvic examination. (But there are times when the doctor does not want to feel the ovaries. In normal postmenopausal women, the ovary shrivels and becomes tiny and difficult, if not impossible, to palpate. If her ovaries are palpable, they may be enlarged by a growing tumor and it is time to worry.)

The prognosis for the cure of early cancer of the ovary is good, with 90 percent cure rates for Stage I. The major problem is that we rarely find patients with Stage I and

II ovarian cancers. The disease has symptoms, but they are vague and often consist only of mild abdominal discomfort, abdominal distension, dyspepsia, and gassiness, for which there seems to be no apparent reason.

Because it is so difficult to detect, I insist that women who are 40 or older return every six months for a pelvic examination to see if there is any change that I can detect with my fingers. If any abnormality is found on pelvic examination, it will be followed up with a sonogram.

In the age group nearing menopause, one-third of ovarian tumors are malignant. But the younger, menstruating woman with an enlarged ovary most likely has only a functional cyst, which will disappear after one or two menstrual cycles. Sometimes a young woman with an enlarged ovary is placed on a birth-control pill to "shut off" her ovary and let it rest. Because it is no longer functioning, it usually gets smaller as the functional cysts disappear. If, however, the enlargement persists after several months, or if the sonogram is suspicious, a laparoscopy should be performed to document the process that is occurring. Remember, 90 percent of ovarian tumors in the under-30 age group are benign.

TUMOR MARKERS IN OVARIAN CANCERS

Because ovarian cancer is so difficult to diagnose in its early stages (at initial diagnosis, two-thirds of the tumors have advanced beyond the ovary), so-called tumor markers are being actively sought. A tumor marker could be any measurable substance in the body that increases or decreases when a tumor is growing. In theory, by measuring changes in the levels of these secondary substances, the physician can get the signal that tumor growth is underway.

Two or three tumor markers are already known, but none signals specifically that the tumor is in the ovaries. One substance, called CEA (carcinoembryonic antigen), is elevated in more than half the women with Stage III ovarian cancer.[6]* Another marker associated with certain types of ovarian tumors is called alpha fetoprotein,[7] and another, called HCG (human chorionic gonadotropin),[8] can also sometimes be used to follow the progress of patients. But we still desperately need to develop a blood test specific to ovarian disease—one that will tell us early that trouble is brewing.

Once ovarian cancer is diagnosed, the ovaries must be surgically removed. Tumor markers are then also helpful in following the progress of the patient, because after the tumor has been removed, the level of these substances falls. Should the tumor recur, it should again produce these same substances. The rise in the amount of these markers would alert the physician that there had been a recurrence of the tumor.

SONOGRAMS

Sometimes when doing pelvic examinations, the doctor is not sure of what he is feeling or even why it feels that way. An ovary may be enlarged, but is it full of cysts, or is there a solid tumor? Could the mass be endometriosis or is it an abscess? When he is unsure, the physician may order a sonogram to diagnose the problem.

Sonography is a form of ultrasound, which has been used for making diagnoses since the early 1950s. Ultrasound uses painless, high-frequency sound waves to "visualize" organs inside the body. The process is much like that used by fishing boats to locate schools of fish. The sound waves bounce off the fish and cause blips on the screen. During the war, enemy submarines were detected in much the same manner.

We are not looking for schools of fish in your tummy, but the principle is the same. The examination begins with the light application of oil to your abdomen. A small probe, called a transducer, held against the skin, sends sound waves

*Stage III ovarian cancer has spread beyond the ovaries.

into the body. The transducer also listens for returning echoes, which have been reflected off the internal organs. These
echoes are converted by the ultrasound's computer into a
visual image on a television-type screen. You can watch the
screen while all this is going on, and the doctor will try
to explain what the pictures mean. Permanent photographs,
film, or videotape records are kept of the examination. One
of the fascinating things about this examination is that the
organs can be watched on the TV as they move. If the
sonogram is taken while you are pregnant, you may see
the heart of your baby beating inside your womb. The baby's
arm or leg motion can also be seen.

There are, of course, many other indications for sonography. Any organ can be outlined. In fact, the heart and
its valves are often checked with this valuable machine.

I have sent many patients with borderline or abnormal
pelvic findings for sonography. An experienced sonographer
can be very helpful in delineating the cause of pelvic pain.
There is no radiation involved with sonography, and aside
from expense, there are no known contraindications. Son-
ograms have helped to confirm diagnoses such as ectopic
pregnancy, cysts of the ovary, and endometriosis. Even when
you are reasonably sure that you know what you are dealing
with, you often get surprises. With sonography to back up
clinical findings, more precise decisions as to whether surgery
is required, or even if an emergency exists, can be made.

COLPOSCOPY

You might one day get a phone call from your doctor's
office and be told that you have a Class II Pap. The doctor
may want to see you again to determine if you have an
infection and give you a cream or some other local therapy.
The Pap test will probably be repeated within six months.
Now, suppose for a moment that you have received a phone
call from your doctor's office telling you that your Pap came
back Class III. Do not panic. Class III does not mean that
you have cancer. It means that there is some area on your

cervix that is shedding abnormal cells. You should return to your doctor, who will repeat your smear. This will confirm that it was really your smear that gave the abnormal results and that no mix-up occurred. This will also give the doctor an opportunity to look at your cervix and try to decide which area or areas are responsible for the abnormality.

Understand that just because you have an abnormal Pap smear, it does not mean that your whole cervix is involved; unless a very widespread process is occurring. Very often only a very tiny area is causing all the fuss. Your doctor may use a colposcope to inspect the area.

The colposcope is a magnifying instrument with a self-contained light. The instrument never touches you; it only serves to illuminate and magnify your cervix when the physician looks through it. As a matter of fact, the magnification is so clear that it is possible to see individual cells and blood-vessel formations. Tiny thickenings and suspicious patterning that would be missed by looking at the cervix with the naked eye are easily seen through the colposcope.

Colposcopy is not a new procedure. It was invented in 1952 by Hans Hinselmann. It has been more widely used in Europe and South America and has only recently gained acceptance in this country. The procedure is neither a substitute for the Pap smear, nor is it a screening method (it cannot be used for screening because of the long time needed for each examination). Its use primarily is to investigate cases where the Pap is reported as abnormal. Because the abnormal area can be visually pinpointed, it can then be exactly biopsied under the magnification of the colposcope. This procedure has stopped the need for multiple biopsies taken "blindly" before the colposcope became available. It has also stopped overtreatment. For example, many women would have had extensive surgery, including conization of the cervix,* were it not for the colposcope. It also sometimes allows minor abnormalities that may occur during pregnancy

---

*Conization, the removal of a large cone-shaped area of cervix, for diagnosis of or therapy for cervical abnormalities.

to be followed visually. This method can spare women from having biopsies performed. For pregnant women, this is especially important, because biopsy often leads to hemorrhage due to the increased blood supply to the area.

The colposcope allows the physician to treat many cervical problems without incurring the risks of anesthesia, hemorrhage, or some other operative complication. It is also useful in the evaluation of benign lesions of the cervix and vagina. Last but not least, it has been the major means of evaluating young women who were exposed to DES (diethylstilbesterol) before they were born. It should be used to visualize the surface of the cervix and vagina in these women whether or not the Pap is normal. It can also be used to easily evaluate a cervix that appears to contain abnormalities, even if the Pap is reported normal.

When a physician looks at a cervix through the colposcope, he usually sees two different areas. One is more red and nearer the opening of the cervix, while the other is shiny and pink and covers the entire cervix, except for the center portion. The area where the two meet is called the transformation zone.

The transformation zone is the active area of the cervix, where cellular change occurs. Here cells from the red inner portion of the cervix (columnar epithelium) actually change into another cell type—squamous epithelium, the cells on the pink, outer portion of the cervix.

The columnar cells lose their tall, columnlike appearance and become flat, platelike, squamous cells. Because the cells in this area are undergoing change and are metabolically active, they are more susceptible to environmental stimuli and carcinogens. Cervical cancer almost always begins in this transformation area.

If the doctor finds a suspicious area, he will probably biopsy it. Having a biopsy taken usually feels something like being pinched. The cervix has very few nerve endings, and so procedures that would be painful to a finger are barely perceptible when done to the cervix. A deep biopsy causes more discomfort, but the discomfort is over in seconds.

If the biopsy indicates less than cancer, the dysplastic area is usually treated with some form of destructive therapy. Heat (hot cautery), cold (freezing the area), electrical destruction, or laser beam are all used for this purpose. These procedures, although they sound awful, take only a few minutes in the physician's office and usually produce no more pain than minimal cramping sensations.

The therapy works because after the abnormal tissue is destroyed, it is replaced by the growth of new, normal tissue. Patients who have had this procedure should be seen again after two months (after two menstrual periods have occurred). A new Pap should be taken, and the patient re-evaluated.

Colposcopy, however, is not infallible. If the abnormal area extends up into the cervical canal or is entirely within the canal, it will be hidden from view, and in this case, further procedures will be necessary. Sometimes acute infections of the cervix will confuse the diagnosis because they cause changes in the appearance of the cervix, which can mask a more insidious process that might be going on underneath in the deeper layers.

If your doctor does not use a colposcope, he will probably do random biopsies at twelve, three, six and nine o'clock on the cervix. The colposcope alleviates the need for multiple biopsies because it enables the physician to see exactly where the problem is and to accomplish a directed biopsy. Often, especially if the lesion is small, the biopsy becomes the cure because it may remove all of the involved area.

If you are scheduled to have a colposcopy, prepare for a fairly long visit. It takes a physician time to look over every square millimeter of cervix and be sure that all is well. You may be bored just lying there. In some offices where many colposcopies are performed, closed-circuit television screens may be set into the ceiling so women can see what the doctor is looking at and ask questions. Most doctors don't have such fancy setups, but you might get lucky.

Because I don't have this apparatus, my patients find themselves looking up at Robert Redford smiling down from the ceiling. He's been quite a conversation piece, and very comforting with his reassuring smile. It sure beats counting squares in the ceiling. I've been looking for a Paul Newman poster for my second examining room, but have yet to find one I want.

Of course, my male patients object to all of this and want Raquel Welch, but as I don't see as many men, they are continually outvoted and will have to be satisfied with the comfort of my smiling face.

ESTROGEN LEVEL

Other procedures may be part of your routine pelvic exam. At the same time that your Pap smear is taken, an estrogen-level test can be performed. The physician simply turns around the Ayre's spatula used for taking the Pap smear and gently passes it over the inner portion of the wall of the vagina. These cells are then smeared on a glass slide, sprayed, and sent to the lab along with your Pap.

The estrogen level (also known as the maturation index or femininity index) provides information on how well your ovaries are functioning. This is not the same information provided by a Pap, which is specifically for malignancy. Vaginal cells are exquisitely sensitive to the effects of estrogen, and by looking at them, it is possible to tell whether your ovaries are producing sufficient amounts of estrogen. In fact, if you are on estrogen-replacement therapy, your doctor can tell whether you are absorbing the estrogen and whether you are receiving a sufficient dose.

Many doctors do not believe in estrogen-level tests, but over the past fifteen years I have found them to be very useful. They're painless to take and add only a second or two to the examination while the patient is already having her Pap done.

I do estrogen-level tests on all my new patients, unless they are on birth-control pills (women on birth-control pills always have the same estrogen level because the pills stop the body's hormonal production and substitute their own constant hormonal levels).

Estrogen-level tests are most useful if they are performed over a period of time on the same patient. I take them in women who have had hysterectomies but whose ovaries have not been removed. A sudden alteration in their estrogen level is a clear warning that something could be wrong with the ovaries. I also follow all of my breast-cancer patients with estrogen-level tests every six months. Primarily, of course, I use estrogen levels to evaluate the hormone-replacement dosage in patients on estrogen-replacement therapy. The estrogen-level test does not provide the fine accuracy of blood tests, but it certainly provides a general indication of the hormonal status of the woman.

Some doctors prefer to do wet smears of the vaginal cells. They take the cells, smear them on a slide, and take a quick overview of which type of cell predominates. The slide is then discarded. I prefer to use a method that treats these slides exactly as a Pap. They are stained and fixed and become permanent records. They are always available if I want to make comparisons months or years later.

I also use estrogen levels to evaluate whether sufficient estrogen is being produced by the patient's ovaries. Estrogen-level tests are repeated as necessary. In young, regularly menstruating women, the test might not be repeated for a few years. A woman who is in her mid to late forties might have the test repeated every six months, because her estrogen level can tie in some of her subjective menopausal symptoms with an actual test result.

For example, I can sometimes tell my patients when they probably will lose their menses and become menopausal. Women approaching menopause often have estrogen levels that gradually decrease. Then there may be a sudden, short-lived increase, and then the "bottom falls out" and the estrogen level rapidly plunges to menopausal levels.

The brief rise in estrogen level happens because the ovary continues to produce estrogen but no longer produces an egg. Consequently, no progesterone is produced. Thus the estrogen level is then influenced only by estrogen and is no longer balanced by progesterone, and this may result in a higher than normal estrogen level. This situation usually does not last long, however, for shortly thereafter, most women note the onset of hot flashes and the slacking of menstruation as the estrogen level rapidly falls. Some women find it reassuring to know that their bodies are undergoing a predictable pattern. I am able to tell patients that they should begin to expect some variation in their menses because of these subtle changes.

VAGINITIS

During a routine pelvic examination, the physician may detect one of the many problems that frequently occur in the pelvic area. Many of these complaints present no bothersome symptoms, so, as in the case of cervical or ovarian cancer, you might not know there is anything wrong until your doctor tells you. Other ailments, however, announce their presence with symptoms unpleasant enough to send you to your physician whether or not it is time for your routine checkup. Among the most common of these complaints are the various forms of vaginitis, which account for nearly one-third of all visits to gynecologists.

The most frequent symptom of vaginitis is a change in the normal vaginal discharge. This may be accompanied by odor and by an annoying, embarrassing itching caused by irritation of the vulva.

Certain factors make vaginitis more likely to occur; you should be watchful for symptoms especially if you take antibiotics or birth-control pills, have a sexual partner who is infected, are menstruating, pregnant, or diabetic. Antibiotics destroy some of the normal bacteria in the vagina, and that allows the infecting organisms to multiply unchecked. It is thought that diabetics may have increased chances of infection because the body's higher sugar level encourages growth of the infecting organism; but this theory is undergoing debate. Menstruation raises the vaginal pH, changing the environment in the vagina from acid to alkaline, and may help foster the growth of organisms other than normal bacteria. Birth-control pills, steroids (cortisone), and pregnancy also increase the chances of infection because they cause other changes in the vaginal chemistry.

The normal adult vagina is resistant to infection because it has an acid pH between 4 and 5, as well as a thick protective cellular covering which is maintained by estrogen. Its particular bacterial population (lactobacilli and corynebacteria) is nourished by glycogen, and the bacteria produce the lactic acid that maintains the normal level of acidity in the vagina. For the young prepubertal girl or the postmenopausal woman who lacks this estrogen protection, vaginitis can be especially troublesome.

Should you notice a bothersome change in your secretions, see your doctor; do not douche for forty-eight hours before your visit, as it will wash away the secretions that are needed for diagnosis. Neither should you use a vaginal contraceptive cream for forty-eight hours, because it will confuse the appearance of the secretions. Also, do not use a tampon because it will remove the diagnostic discharge.

Normal secretions are usually white, clear, or gray, and have an acid pH (usually less than 5). Abnormal secretions may look thick and curdy, like cottage cheese, or may be gray-green and runny, or any variation in between. A doctor cannot make a correct diagnosis of infection just by looking at the secretions. Attempts to do so lead to wrong diagnoses in 50 percent of cases. Getting the correct diagnosis is very important, because proper treatment for each infection type is quite different, and the wrong treatment can make matters even worse. Also it is possible to have more than one type of infection at a time.

Accurate diagnoses are easily made by taking some of

the secretion on a cotton applicator, adding it to a normal saline (balanced salt) solution, placing a couple of drops on a glass slide, and viewing it under a microscope. There the three most common causes of vaginitis display their unique characteristic patterns: *Candida* (monilia) is a fungus, *Trichomonas* is a tiny motile organism, and *Hemophilus vaginitis* is a bacteria.

Candida Vaginitis

Candida is the most common type of vaginitis and one which may not necessarily be sexually transmitted. It is present in the body of almost everyone at some time and small amounts are probably present in the normal vagina. It can remain quiescent for years, only to become active at the most inopportune moment. It produces intense itching, especially at night, and there may be a burning sensation during sexual intercourse or after voiding. Symptoms may range from mild irritation to severe swelling and redness that involve the vulva and rectal area. Discharge is often thick and white-yellow and cottage cheese-like. However, little or no discharge may be noted. Men with *Candida* often have burning and itching also. But a man may be totally symptom free and still have *Candida* in his semen or on his penis.

Candida is best diagnosed under the microscope, where its characteristic yeast buds and threadlike elements can be seen. This infection also shows up in an acid pH (from 4.0 to 4.5).

There are several vaginal creams (such as miconazole, clotrimazole, or nystatin) on the market to cure this problem. Most of them are used for seven days, inserted into the vagina at bedtime. If the itching and swelling of the vulva are intolerable, a cortisone cream applied to the labia is soothing and reduces the inflammation. If the infection is especially stubborn, it may be necessary to continue the therapy longer or take pills to kill the *Candida* that may be living in the gastrointestinal tract. The infection, if persistent, may also be a clue that the patient is diabetic.

Trichomonas Vaginitis

Trichomonas vaginitis is caused by a protozoan parasite that is transmitted by sexual relations. Some women who harbor this organism have no symptoms; many have a profuse gray-green discharge that causes itching, discomfort, and odor. Seen under a microscope, the *Trichomonas* organisms are a little bigger than the white blood cells on the same slide. They can easily be spotted because they move in an erratic dance in and out among the white blood cells and other debris on the slide. Sometimes I invite my patients to peer into the microscope to see them. This has a significant impact on them and usually guarantees that they take all their medication. None of my patients cares to share her body with such frantic little creatures. "Trich" can also be diagnosed on Pap smears or suspected from the little red "strawberry marks" that it causes on the cervix or vaginal wall. It exists in a pH between 5 and 7.

The treatment for "trich" is Flagyl (metronidazole), a pill taken three times per day for seven days by both sexual partners. Although only 20 percent of infected males have symptoms, it is important that the male also be treated, because he can reinfect the woman who has just been cured. While you are taking Flagyl, do not drink any alcoholic beverages, for even a tiny amount can make you violently ill.

Hemophilus Vaginitis

Hemophilus vaginitis is a bacterial infection that is frequently confused with *Trichomonas vaginitis* because the discharges look alike. Under the microscope, however, an experienced physician can spot the "clue cell," a bacteria-laden vaginal-lining cell. If no clue cells are seen, the slide can be stained for more specific identification of the bacteria, or cultures can be sent to a laboratory for analysis.

Hemophilus is a common venereal disease, although it may produce few symptoms because the bacteria do not invade the tissue but remain near the surface. Men rarely have complaints, although they carry and transmit the bacteria easily.

In women, *Hemophilus* produces odor and large amounts of grayish discharge, but often it is not irritating or itchy to a woman. Not uncommonly it is the husband's complaints of odor rather than the woman's own irritation that send her to the doctor's office.

Hemophilus is transmitted sexually, but a woman can become infected even without having had sex recently, since an episode may be just a flareup of an old infection that has been present for a long time without showing symptoms. It is best treated with antibiotics (given to both partners) or Flagyl. However, because of possible adverse side effects from Flagyl—it has been implicated as a possible carcinogen—and because this infection is not very serious, it can also be treated locally with creams or antibiotics, especially when there is no monogamous relationship and multiple reinfections are likely.

Atrophic Vaginitis

Atrophic vaginitis is the term for changes that occur in the vaginal tissue when estrogen support is lost due to menopause, surgical removal of the ovaries, or radiation therapy of the ovaries. The vagina becomes thin and loses its normal anatomical folds and secretions. It becomes dry and tends to bleed easily. And it becomes susceptible to a mixed bacterial infection that causes an irritating discharge. Tenderness and itching make life miserable for the woman with this problem. Estrogen, taken either orally or as a vaginal cream, will give her relief by making the vaginal tissues more resistant to bacterial and other infections.

Herpes

Herpes type II is five times as prevalent as syphilis and rivals gonorrhea for the number-one spot among venereal diseases. A first infection with herpes is not easily forgotten. And like its cousin herpes type I, which causes cold sores, once the virus has infected you, it stays forever. (Herpes type I used to be described as occurring above the belly button, while herpes type II occurred below, but since the so-called sexual revolution, the two types have appeared in upside-down locations.) Since herpes is a virus, and since few antiviral drugs are available at this time, there is no cure for this painful condition. Much research on a great variety of medications is currently taking place, however, so a cure may soon be found.

Genital herpes begins as red, blisterlike structures. Usually there are several lesions on the vulva, but the vagina or cervix can also be involved. The lesions break down in twenty-four to forty-eight hours, ulcerate, and become small, tender, shallow ulcers. These ulcers last three to fourteen days and then heal without scarring. If the lesions are located on the cervix, there is often a heavy discharge.

The first infection that occurs after exposure to the virus is the worst. It can cause fever, lethargy, swelling of the lymph nodes in the groin, and swelling of the vulva. If the lesions are close to the outlet of the bladder, urination may be impossible because of the pain. Such patients must be admitted to hospitals for catheterization.

Like the fever blisters that occur time and time again on the mouth when you have a cold or are out in the sun, *Herpes genitalis* also recurs. It may recur when your body defenses are down and you are not feeling well, and in women, it most often occurs premenstrually. The virus migrates up into the nerve root and remains dormant until conditions are right, and then it migrates down the nerve again to the skin and begins a new series of blisters and annoyance. Recurrent herpes attacks, however, are less painful and less noticeable than the first. They also last for a much shorter time. Nevertheless, the lesions are just as infective. Indeed, there is some thought that people who have herpes may shed the virus all the time, whether or not lesions are present.

There is much speculation that herpes infection of the cervix might lead to cervical cancer. For safety's sake, a woman with genital herpes should be sure to have routine Pap smears.

A major problem exists with pregnant woman, who can

spread the disease to their newborn infants. This infection can sometimes end in death or brain damage to the child. Any woman who has had *herpes genitalis* should alert her physician so that he can observe her carefully. If active lesions are present at the time of labor, her child will be delivered by cesarean section.

Chlamydia Trachomatitis

Chlamydia is a bacterial infection, although the infecting organism itself may be a transition between virus and bacteria. This disease, only recently recognized, is also currently being called the most common sexually transmitted disease. (As you must now realize, several diseases are trying to achieve this distinction.) If a man harbors the organism, then it will usually appear in the cervical cultures of 70 percent of his female partners. In woman, chlamydia is thought to contribute to Pelvic Inflammatory Disease (PID), and currently it is also being implicated in cervical cancer, although the final word is not yet in. Interestingly, it is now also being implicated as a possible cause of Reiter's syndrome, an unusual arthritis that involves the joints, eyes, and mucous membranes. It seems likely that in certain genetically susceptible individuals, this arthritis might be precipitated by such an infectious process (chlamydia).

Most women, however, have no symptoms. Most men do, because in men, chlamydia produces urethritis, a watery discharge and a slight burning of the urethra.

Commonly, chlamydia and gonorrhea are found together. Chlamydia, however, has a longer incubation period and takes longer to appear. As a result, some patients who show symptoms of gonorrhea are treated with penicillin (which does not affect chlamydia), seem to do well, and then develop symptoms again. The chances are that these symptoms are not a recurrence of gonorrhea but the first signs of chlamydia, which has not been touched by the gonorrhea treatment.

In women, an acute infection of the cervix is usually taken as a sign of chlamydia by an examining physician. However, the organism can be identified only by means of growing laboratory cultures, a long process usually not available in most doctors' offices. Instead, your physician usually will first test for gonorrhea by culture and smears, and if these tests prove negative, he may treat you for chlamydia, if your cervix looks suspicious. The antibiotic recommended for this infection is tetracycline, given for two or three weeks. As usual, both partners should be treated.

VENEREAL DISEASE

Venereal Disease (VD) is named after Venus, the goddess of love, because it is a group of contagious diseases contracted through sexual intercourse. In the United States, venereal diseases are spreading at an astonishing rate: one new case every fifteen seconds. Gonorrhea is one of the two most common and most serious venereal diseases. (The other, of course, is syphilis.) Gonorrhea ranks second only to flu among the reportable diseases in this country, and it is suspected that 80 to 85 percent of the cases are never reported. (Syphilis ranks fourth in this category.) It is most prevalent among teenagers and young adults. Most females with VD (85 percent) don't even know they have it, and about 20 percent of males who have it are also without symptoms. Over one million people in the United States have the disease and don't know about it.

Widespread use of condoms, which protect from infection, can significantly reduce the incidence of VD. In Sweden, where the use of condoms has been officially encouraged, gonorrhea has declined, while in the United States, the use of the pill and the IUD have increased the rate of contagion. In addition, a recent study has confirmed an old-fashioned tale, demonstrating that it is possible, *in theory*, to contract gonorrhea from a toilet seat or contaminated toilet paper, although so far no instances of such nonsexual transmission have actually been documented.[9]

The worst consequence of gonorrhea is that it damages the fallopian tubes, causing women to become sterile. The tubes become scarred, so that the egg can no longer be transported from the ovary into the uterus. Or the scarring prevents the growing fertilized egg from passing into the uterus, causing an ectopic or tubal pregnancy.

This damage can be prevented if the gonorrhea is treated in time. Unfortunately, since the disease often causes no symptoms, some women realize they have it too late or only when a partner develops signs of infection. In the United States, between fifty thousand and eighty thousand young women are robbed of fertility in this way every year.[10] Other women, not knowing for weeks or months that anything is wrong, unwittingly become carriers, infecting their partners and spreading the disease further.

The symptoms of gonorrhea, when they do appear, are varied and deceptively mild. There may be a yellow-green discharge that causes little itching. The discharge may be minimal, and although the average incubation period for the disease is two to eight days, the menses may easily mask the discharge and the onset of infection. There may be some minor variation in flow or menstrual discomfort. (Interestingly, gonorrhea can also occur in women who have had hysterectomies. These women have a vaginal infection and often an infection of the urethra, the outlet of the bladder.)

If the gonococcus (the organism causing gonorrhea) works its way up into the fallopian tubes, pelvic inflammatory disease ensues. The disease process produces considerable pelvic discomfort and a low-grade fever; and the doctor's pelvic examination may be painful because the pelvic organs are infected and inflamed.

If the disease progresses further, the bacteria may invade the bloodstream and cause arthritis, which is usually accompanied by skin lesions.

There is now a blood test for gonorrhea, but it has specific limitations and uses; because the test is new, there is some controversy as to just how accurate and useful it will be. (Three manufacturers in the United States have been granted FDA approval for such blood tests.) The test, specifically designed for screening populations of asymptomatic women, is especially helpful in areas where pelvic examinations are not routinely done. However, it cannot be used in patients with prior infections of gonorrhea or meningococcal meningitis, and it is not for women who already have symptoms and need cultures taken.

It is possible that soon there may be a vaccine available to prevent gonorrhea. The vaccine will most likely give additional protection against sister bacteria which are known to cause some forms of meningitis.

If you think you have been exposed to gonorrhea, it is essential that you get to a doctor. Even if you have no symptoms, you must see your doctor if a male partner is diagnosed as having gonorrhea. Other sex partners must also be told, so that they do not reinfect you or spread the disease to others.

Luckily gonorrhea can be cured with antibiotics. Usually it is treated with injectable penicillin or with other antibiotics given orally. Since there is no absolute guarantee that you will be cured by the therapy, you will be asked to return for a follow-up visit. Remember, no immunity or resistance to the disease is acquired by having had gonorrhea. It can be contracted many times, and each time it is equally dangerous.

New laws state that doctors and VD clinics need not notify parents of minors, and treatment will be given without their consent or knowledge. In California, anyone over the age of 12 can seek care for venereal disease without parental consent, and the physician is barred from informing the child's parents.

Syphilis

Syphilis is probably the most serious venereal disease of all, because in its late stages, it destroys many body organs such as the brain, liver, bone, and heart valves. We rarely if ever see late syphilis today, because doctors are more aware of the early stages and are able to treat them before the disease advances.

The first or primary stage consists of a *painless* single sore although there may be discomfort from chafing of the lesions by underclothing. In men, it is usually on the penis, but it may also be on the mouth, finger, or other extragenital area. In women, these lesions may be on the labia or hidden within the vagina or cervix and never noticed. These lesions usually appear about three weeks after infection and heal without treatment in a few weeks. Lymph nodes in the groin may become swollen and tender some seven to ten days after development of the chancre (sore).

Blood tests for syphilis may be negative during the first three to four weeks, but infected material can be taken from the chancre itself and tested by a procedure called a darkfield examination.

Without treatment, lesions of secondary syphilis usually appear after the primary chancre has healed. These lesions consist of a red-brown, slightly raised rash, often resembling a viral rash but persisting for weeks. Other skin lesions may develop involving the entire body or just the palms of the hands and the soles of the feet. These lesions appear bilaterally—that is, on *both* hands or feet—on symmetrical areas. These areas may itch, though they usually don't. Moist, flat, raised areas may appear in the anogenital area; lymph nodes may enlarge without becoming tender; and hair may be lost near the scalp margins and the eyebrows.

By that time, the infecting organism will have spread throughout the body by way of the bloodstream. A low-grade fever may be present. The blood tests will then be positive. And because there are so many lesions containing infective organisms, secondary syphilis is the most contagious stage of the disease.

In late-stage syphilis, the patient no longer has a rash or chancre. There are no symptoms. This phase may last from a few months to several years. Infectivity decreases with time, and by the fourth year, the ability to transmit the disease is minimal. Nevertheless, a pregnant woman with late syphilis can still transmit the disease to her child, even after she has had the disease for many years. (That is why all pregnant women are tested for syphilis and treated if the tests prove positive.) About 30 percent of patients (of both sexes) with late syphilis go on to develop serious destruction of body organs.

I could go on and on, for there are more diseases that are sexually transmitted than you could count on all your fingers and toes. Chancroid, lymphogranuloma venereum, and granuloma inguinale are some of the minor venereal diseases. Hepatitis B can also be sexually passed.

If, after you read this chapter, sex seems to be a little more serious and less casual—it is. Sexual activity is the source of most of the diseases that affect the pelvic area. Unfortunately, we still have no immunization for VD. We have no drug prophylaxis. The only way to avoid infection is to avoid exposure. Abstinence, of course, will do. Keeping down the number of sexual contacts will help. Currently, however, condoms offer the only known effective prophylaxis against the transmission of herpes, gonorrhea, *Trichomonas*, and so on. They also prevent possibly cancer-causing semen from coming in contact with the cervix. Combined with a contraceptive foam, which has antibacterial and some antiviral activity, they provide your best chance of remaining in good health, especially if your sexual partner is new or not yours alone.

Other problems of the pelvic area, however, are not sexually transmitted (so far as we know), but, like ovarian cancer, they may be even more deadly. So even women who are celibate or who confine their sexual relationships to other women must protect themselves by regular, routine pelvic exams and Pap tests.

Luckily, most of the ailments of the pelvic area are easily detected and fairly easily cured. And some of the worst of them, such as cervical cancer, can be prevented by following routine prophylactic procedures and seeking routine physician care.

There is wisdom in the old advice: if you can't be good, be careful. And here's some advice your mother probably never gave you: if you are not in a stable relationship with a disease-free partner, carry your own condoms (so that he never has *that* excuse). And whether you experience unpleasant symptoms or not, visit regularly a physician you trust to examine you thoroughly and inform you fully about the state of your pelvic area. It's your pelvis, and unfortunately it can be the site of endless "female" troubles. But with the help of a few precautions and a good physician, you can keep your pelvic area in healthy, normal condition.

CHAPTER 8

Body Housekeeping

Precious little has been written to inform women how to care for their bodies, especially those portions below the belly button. And there is virtually no one to talk to about basic female hygiene. Most of the information we have is simply a jumble of old-fashioned tales and modern-day mythology. The medical world is equally confused because most gynecologists happen to be men who have no first-hand knowledge of these matters and make little effort to find anything out. As a result, most of the advice on body care that women usually receive from their gynecologists is pure gibberish. I will present here the information that I pass on to my patients for your consideration, and you can use it or not, as you see fit.

HOW TO TAKE CARE OF YOUR BOTTOM

Most of my patients are convinced that proper care of the genital area requires plenty of soap and water. Should they develop an irritation in this area, they try to correct it by vigorous rubbing with a bar of soap. Nothing could make matters worse. Soap is generally very alkaline and drying, so you should never rub a bar of soap over your vulvar area or let soap get into your vagina. Rather, rub the bar of soap into the pubic hairs and put it down. Then take the bubbles that you have made and spread them down over the vulva and wash with them. Don't use a washcloth. Use your fingers, for only in that way can you separate the labia and clean well between the folds. If you usually shower instead of taking a bath, thorough rinsing can be difficult; and rinsing is actually more important than washing. Women would have fewer problems if they simply used less soap and more water. One of the best ways to rinse the area is to purchase a French shower or some type of shower head that connects to the wall via a long hose. It even lets you wash and rinse your bottom without taking a full shower and without disturbing your makeup or hairdo. And it is much more effective than using a deodorant spray. In most cases, the odor that is detectable after a warm day (especially when one has been wearing pantyhose) is produced by a small residue of urine, which it is impossible to wipe completely from the vulva, plus some perspiration. Washing the area, unlike using spray deodorants, does not just cover up the odor but gets rid of its source.

The shower apparatus, however, must never be used for douching. The water stream is too forceful and could be dangerous.

If you do not have a French shower or it is not possible to shower, a large cotton ball soaked with warm water can be used effectively for cleansing the vulva after urination. If you like, you may then spray on a deodorant lightly, *if* you are not sensitive to such sprays. Most women don't need deodorants if they clean the area properly. (Europeans have solved this problem by installing bidets in their bathrooms. If you are lucky enough to have one, enjoy it).

Toilet paper is something that also can cause problems. Some women develop irritations because they are sensitive to perfumed toilet paper. Others are sensitive to colored paper. (Colored toilet tissue is also less biodegradable.) So to be on the safe side, plain white toilet paper is probably the best for the family.

When using toilet paper for cleansing the rectal area, wipe the rectal area backward, away from the vaginal opening, to prevent infection. Ideally, cleansing should be accomplished after bowel movements, especially in women who have rectal irritation. The French shower or cotton balls may conveniently be used for this purpose. Commercial products such as Tucks are also available.

DOUCHING

Douching is another taboo subject, as menstrual pain was a little while ago. Little is written about it and less is spoken. I sent an article on douching to one of the more liberal women's magazines some years ago and received it back with a rejection that stated, "We don't print that sort of article!" Most women do not talk about douching, even with other women. It's as though it were some kind of deep, dark, dirty secret. A few years ago at a medical meeting, I tried to engage a well-known female endocrinologist in a discussion about douching. She became very defensive and said, "It's completely unnecessary." And she left me standing alone while she sought out more compatible company.

I'm sure that my woman-doctor acquaintance took umbrage at my question because she felt that admitting that you douche is like admitting that you are dirty. I don't see it that way at all. I don't think that anyone *must* douche. On the other hand, if you want to—if it makes you feel better, cleaner, more anything—then do it.

Douching is not really a medical matter at all. Yet for years, physicians have been telling their patients that it is. Interestingly, about half those physicians told women that they should not douche since the vagina cleans itself and douching can ruin the natural cleansing action, while the other half urged that douching is indeed necessary and must be performed according to explicit instructions. That such a divergence of opinion exists leads to only one conclusion: male physicians and male douche manufacturers don't really know.

Personally, I feel that douching is no more a medical problem than brushing your teeth is. I have scanned the medical literature from 1968 on and found only five or six articles on the subject, and the only maladies connected with it worldwide were a total of nine cases of abdominal infection (peritonitis) resulting from air insufflation during douching. However, whether or not it has been "prescribed" by a physician, douching is a reality for more than half the female population of this country.

Some women are simply more fastidious than others. Others feel it necessary to douch after their menses in order to get rid of retained blood-breakdown products. Perhaps these women are more rapidly cleansing their bodies of substances that provide good culture media for unwanted infections. Some women douche after having sexual intercourse, because if they don't, they are annoyed by semen leaking onto the bed sheets, while others never have this happen and don't douche at all. Remember that as long as the douche solution is properly diluted, you can do little harm by frequent douching. If a woman has sexual intercourse every day and wants to douche afterward, that's fine. If her vagina is up to having intercourse every day, it's up to douching every day.

Even in early pregnancy, douching is safe unless it is a high-risk pregnancy or the patient has a cervical abnormality. The postmenopausal woman who is on estrogen therapy can douche safely because she has a healthy, resilient vagina. However, the postmenopausal woman who is not on hormone replacement might injure her more fragile tissues.

Keep in mind that mechanical cleansing is the greatest benefit of douching. If you have ever had to apply a vaginal cream for an infection each night before bed, you know that the cream tends to become more fluid and leak down and out for most of the next day. To feel secure, you must often wear a pad. The next night, you are supposed to apply a second inserter full of cream into your vagina. After a few days and nights, the amount of accumulated cream becomes prodigious, and the constant leakage and the pad become irritating. Your directions almost never include any advice about douching away the accumulated cream. Yet would you take care of an infection on your arm by applying one coat of antibacterial cream on top of another without washing or at least wiping it with peroxide between applications? Why should you treat an infection in your vagina differently?

If you have vaginitis, you already have excessive secretion of pus, mucus, dead cellular debris, and bacteria. You should insert the cream at bedtime and douche it out in the morning when you wake up. That way you will be fresh, clean, non-itchy, and nondripping for the day. At night, simply reapply the cream to the clean area. I always advise patients to douche out their creams the following morning, but I have never yet had a patient whose gynecologist instructed her to douche out the old remains of a vaginal cream.

Someday a study should be done of a group of women who douche regularly after intercourse and a group who don't to see if either group has a preponderance of vaginitis, abnormal Paps, herpes vaginitis, or venereal disease. Marital status and number of sexual partners would have to be accounted for, of course. It may turn out that while douching is basically not a medical matter, there are some medical reasons, which may benefit women, that doctors have completely overlooked. Furthermore, we know that cervical cancer is more prevalent among sexually active women with multiple partners, or who have herpes or other infections. Because washing viruses off your hands is the best way to protect yourself from catching colds, douching after intercourse to wash away viruses and semen from the cervix may help prevent cervical cancer.

What kind of douche apparatus should you buy?

If you are at all serious about douching, buy a douche bag. Disposable douches are too expensive and do not contain enough fluid to do the job adequately. Besides, you do not have to be a mathematical genius to measure out a quarter-teaspoon of douche preparation or a tablespoon of white vinegar into a quart of water. In the long run, you will be much better off with your own equipment. Possibly I should emphasize the words *your own.* Never share a douche bag with anyone else, even your sister or your mother.

There is some little variation in douche equipment. Each contains a bag to hold the water and douche preparation. Each has a nozzle which is to be inserted into the vagina. The major difference is that some douche bags come with a hose that connects it to the nozzle, while other types have no hose. One of these has a valve through which the nozzle is attached directly to the bag; others have screw-on nozzles.

The douche bag that has a hose is probably easier to use. (It is designed so that it can also be used as an enema bag. A second, tiny nozzle is provided for this purpose.) The only disadvantage with this type of bag is that the hose must be drained before it can be stored. If it bothers you to see a douche bag hanging in the bathroom, buy the type without the hose. It can be neatly packed away in its case immediately after use, but it has its disadvantages as well. The biggest one in one model is that because of the placement of the valve, the bag has to be jammed up into the faucet to fill it. You must have a proper-size faucet, and even then, you should expect to get yourself and the ceiling of the bathroom sprayed from time to time if the bag slips on the faucet. This can be quite a rude awakening, especially at 2 A.M. The startled yell that accompanies the unexpected bath can also be disconcerting to your partner. In addition to this fault, like all of the others, it is poorly designed in that it cannot be cleaned between uses.

I have never recommended using a foul, medicinal-smelling douche. There is no reason to use such a product. Nor do I routinely recommend douches containing iodine, because they may produce allergic reactions, change the vaginal bacteria, or cause problems from the absorption of iodine. Iodine-containing douches are especially dangerous if you are pregnant, for the excess iodine will be absorbed by the fetus. So read your labels.

Instead I sometimes recommend douche preparations that contain detergents or wetting agents which help emulsify vaginal secretions and liquefy small particulate matter so the douche solution can carry it all away. The old, time-tested douche solution of white vinegar and water is also effective, and if you are lazy, you can buy it already mixed in an offensive, strong-smelling disposable form that sells for nearly $1.

The most important points are that the water you use should always be lukewarm, never hot, and the preparation should be mixed according to the directions so that it is not too concentrated. If it is made too strong, the ingredients could irritate your tissues. And some douches, prepared in a more concentrated form than the directions call for, will bubble you right out of the bathroom.

Prone to Douche?

For years, women have been instructed to douche in the most unsanitary, uncomfortable position imaginable: lying down in a bathtub.

Some four to five years ago, when I was reading the labels on douche products and looking at the illustrations that showed how douching must be accomplished in the bathtub, I became extremely annoyed that such archaic methods should be perpetuated, not only by physicians but by the douche manufacturers themselves. Thinking that if I could get one of the manufacturers to rewrite their douching instructions, possibly other manufacturers might follow suit, I called the vice-president of one of the companies. He invited me to lunch at a New York City business club. Lunch turned out to be a waste of time. The company was not about to change their instructions. They wrote me a follow-up letter that said they would consider changing the instructions and would contact their "experts." From time to time, I've reviewed their instructions. Years have passed, and so far nothing has changed.

Consequently, I instruct every one of my patients to pay no attention to the package insert that tells them how to douche. I explain that those douching instructions are from the Dark Ages.

It is not pleasant to put your naked, bony back against a cold, hard bathtub bottom, especially in the morning while you are racing to get to work. First you have dirty water trickling down your legs and buttocks. Then, as soon as you sit or stand up, the rest of the fluid which has accumulated in the vagina runs out, which is a pretty good reason to refill the tub and bathe again.

Any woman can douche much more quickly and effectively while sitting on the toilet and can perfectly and adequately cleanse her vagina in no more than two minutes. Simply compress the vaginal lips together around the douche nozzle for a few seconds while administering the douche solution. This will cause the vagina to fill to the top. Then release the labia to allow the douche water to gush back out into the toilet bowl. Repeat this two or three times until the quart of douche liquid is used up.

Any concern about the vagina not being adequately cleansed by this method is misplaced. We know that the vaginal wall is folded, and the traditional worry has been that unless the fluid is administered while lying horizontally, the water would never reach the top of the vagina nor would the vaginal folds get adequately cleansed. Well, when a woman is seated and the vaginal lips are compressed while the douche solution is flowing in, the vagina rapidly fills up. What's more, the vagina is in a much better position to empty and does so much more rapidly, thereby taking more debris and loosened sediment along. While the vaginal lips are compressed, the vaginal wall is adequately ballooned out for effective cleansing of and between the folds. In the lying-down position, the douche solution trickles out slowly over a longer time period, allowing settling out of infected material in the upper vagina. In a sitting position, the downward slant of the vagina and gravity create a faster flow of water out of the vagina and provide a better mechanical cleansing.

Another concern that people express from time to time

is whether douching produces any lasting changes in vaginal pH. A study by Glynn[1] in which women douched daily for a month with a variety of solutions, both acid and alkaline, showed no long-term changes in vaginal pH as measured electronically with a Beckman pH meter. Nor were mucosal changes detected in a microscopic analysis. So whether an acid or an alkaline douche is used, the vaginal pH returns to its former level within half an hour after douching. Just as you wouldn't worry about what effect acid or alkaline foods have on the tissues of your mouth (which is made up of similar cells), there is no evidence suggesting that you need to worry about the mild pH of douche solutions. Semen deposited in the vagina changes the vaginal pH for approximately two hours. (I have yet to hear a ban on intercourse suggested by my colleagues who intimidate patients about the perils of douche products that change the vaginal pH.)

So although there is no reason to feel that you must douche, there is also no reason to feel that douching will be harmful to you. Properly done in the sitting position, it need not even be uncomfortable or time consuming. But whether to douche is up to you.

TAMPONS

Tampons were used as early as the second century by Roman, Egyptian, and Babylonian women. Yet in this sophisticated twentieth century, many women have rather old-fashioned ideas about them.

Despite the extensive advertising of tampons, many women are still in the dark about how they actually work. Some women do not use tampons because they are afraid that they will put them in wrong and harm themselves or that the tampon will get lost and migrate into the abdomen. Others complain that they tried once, it hurt, and they never tried again.

Actually, when a tampon is properly placed, it cannot be felt at all. That's one of the nicest things about tampons.

You are completely free of napkins, free of the sensations of draining fluids, free from chafing from blood accumulated on the vulva and hair, free from the slight odor that begins when blood is exposed to the air. (For the most part, used tampons have no odor because the blood has not been exposed to the air.)

After a tampon is inserted, any discomfort is almost certainly due to the tampon not being inserted far enough. Pushing the tampon in a little further will end the discomfort. Keep in mind that it is not possible to insert a tampon too far. The vagina is a closed tube except for the tiny opening into the uterus, which is much too small for a tampon to pass through; so a tampon that is pushed in deeply can go only as far in as the depth of the vagina and no further.

Patients sometimes worry that the tampon will block the flow of blood and prevent it from coming out, but tampons have been designed to absorb the flow, not block it. They are made from a variety of materials, and the percentages of the various materials change from junior to regular to super tampons. The materials and their proportion depend on how absorbent the tampon is supposed to be.

You should try to use the appropriate-size tampon for the amount of flow you expect that day. If you expect a heavy flow, then a super or superplus tampon is appropriate. As the flow lessens, you should use a regular or junior tampon because the superabsorbent ones may be more closely associated with the development of Toxic Shock Syndrome. And, since these super sizes will not become saturated on days of spotting or light flow, they will tend to stick to the vaginal wall a little and be harder to remove. Because superplus tampons absorb so well, they can actually pull fluid from the vaginal cells and cause irritation and drying. So it is best to use smaller sizes on days with less flow. And because of the recent problems with Toxic Shock Syndrome, you might be better off using napkins at some convenient time during your flow, such as in the beginning, when you are only spotting, and after the heavy flow is over, when you are only bleeding lightly. Some women have elected to use napkins at night to decrease the time of continuous tampon use.

Some tampons come with inserters and others do not; the choice between them depends upon individual preference. Tampons without inserters are smaller and easier to carry in a small pocketbook; and, of course, they have no inserters to be disposed of afterward. (Cardboard inserters are biodegradable and can be flushed down the toilet, but plastic inserters will clog plumbing.) Many women who have trouble placing the tampon prefer to use inserters. You should try both kinds to determine which you like better. Deodorant tampons may make the bathroom smell nice, but the deodorant is superfluous and may even produce an allergic reaction.

Should young girls try tampons? Most definitely yes. It is the rare young woman who has a hymen so tight that a junior tampon cannot pass through. (It is possible, however, and if you have a persistent problem, ask your doctor why.) Young women, because of their constant physical activity, will find tampons especially convenient to use.

One word of caution: though tampons may be excellent for catching menstrual flow, either used alone or with an accompanying napkin, they should not be used chronically for absorbing vaginal discharge. Using a tampon when there is no bleeding but only slight excess discharge can irritate the vaginal tissues and contribute to your general discomfort.

TOXIC SHOCK SYNDROME (TSS)

TSS was first described in 1978 by Dr. James Todd, a pediatrician. The illness occurred in several children who had high fever, headache, sore throat, diarrhea, and a sunburn-type rash. The children's lab findings indicated abnormal kidney and liver function, and all of them developed low blood pressure that was difficult to normalize. One of the children died. The others experienced peeling of the skin on their hands and feet seven or eight days after the beginning of their illness.

In the second half of 1979, several women were hospitalized in Wisconsin with symptoms similar to those described by Todd. Six of the women were menstruating at the time they became ill. One young girl, however, had not yet begun to menstruate.

Because of the close geographical proximity of these cases, the Department of Health in Wisconsin began to survey the state for further cases. The Minnesota Department of Health reported a similar occurrence and also began a statewide survey. The national Center for Disease Control (CDC) in Atlanta was alerted, and a nationwide effort was made to collect data on women with the disease.

TSS made newspaper headlines across the United States in 1980. Healthy, menstruating women were suddenly struck down by a serious, sometimes deadly illness. Those women who used tampons seemed especially vulnerable.

Rely tampons, the newest brand on the market, came under particularly close scrutiny. When it became clear that more cases of TSS were related to the use of Rely than to other brands of tampons, the manufacturer voluntarily withdrew Rely from the market.

With all the publicity surrounding TSS, there was a 15% decline in tampon use from July 1980 to January 1981. By January 1981, there were 941 confirmed cases of TSS and 73 deaths in the United States, but the number of cases showed a definite downward trend from a high of 106 cases in September 1980, decreasing to 58 in October and to only 32 in December. The researchers at the Center for Disease Control believed that the decline in TSS was related to the withdrawal of Rely tampons from the market.

The disease, however, has occurred with the use of every brand of tampon. One case has also been confirmed in a woman using sanitary napkins and another in a woman using sea sponges. It is important that you not become complacent about TSS simply because Rely is no longer available. You should watch for signs and symptoms of the disease, especially if you use tampons throughout your entire cycle.

There is evidence that TSS is related to continuous tampon use and the CDC has recommended that women who use tampons, and would like to decrease the risk of TSS, use them intermittently. That would mean using napkins when flow is light, or alternating with napkins during the night.

You should know the symptoms and signs of TSS. *If you are menstruating, using tampons, and experiencing symptoms similar to those that follow, you should contact your physician. You should also immediately remove your tampon.* Although symptoms may begin at any time during or immediately following menstruation, the average onset is the fourth day of the menstrual flow.

fever over 102 degrees
dizziness or low blood pressure upon assuming a standing
   position
confusion, disorientation accompanied by low blood pressure
rash over most of the body, or confined to the palms and
   soles (rash is diffuse, often looks like the skin is flushed
   or sunburned; rash may rarely appear as tiny purple spots
   that do not blanch)
peeling occurs on the hands and feet approximately one
   to two weeks after the onset of the illness
nausea and vomiting
diarrhea
muscular aches and pains
redness of the eyes, mouth, or vagina
abnormal laboratory findings for liver and kidney functions
decreased platelet counts
negative results for other infectious diseases

Many causes of TSS have been postulated. According to Kathryn Shands, M.D., of the CDC, studies show that the incidence of the disease is *not* influenced by the following factors: frequency of sexual intercourse, frequency of sexual intercourse during menstruation, length of time between tampon changes, amount or duration of menstrual flow, use of superabsorbent tampons, or personal hygiene practices. It has been noted, however, that women who had TSS seemed to use birth-control methods less often.[2]

Clearly, we don't know why TSS develops in some women. Tampons, of course, are widely used by women in the United States and the actual incidence of TSS is very low. It approximates 6.2 cases per 100,000 menstruating women per year.[3] Certainly, there are additional factors besides the use of tampons that cause TSS.

TAKING CARE OF YOU

Throughout this book, I have tried to put in plain English some technical, medical information so that you can be a better-educated consumer of professional health care. But I am first of all a family doctor, so in conclusion, I would like to give you a little family-doctor advice about taking care of yourself. That means getting down to some simple concerns, for all the developments of modern medicine may do you little good if you disregard basic health care. On that subject, our mothers and grandmothers had a lot to say. How often have you been told, "Get some rest," or, "So eat a little something"? Medically speaking, it's good advice.

Diet

Most people take better care of their cars than their bodies. They would never dream of running a car without oil, because they know the engine would quickly be ruined. Yet they think nothing of running their bodies all day without food.

It is a funny thing that none of my overweight patients ever eats breakfast. In fact, most of them never eat lunch, either. Instead, they eat a "supper" that lasts all night. Women are especially notorious for practically fasting all day, then stuffing everything in sight into their mouths when they reach home after work. No wonder; they're literally starving. I believe that people who eat only one meal per day cannot metabolize it properly. Because their bodies are conditioned to starve during the day, they tend to store up food energy as fat rather than preparing it for immediate burning, as the body would do if it had sufficient amounts of food throughout the day. If people who eat only one big meal a day divided that food into three small meals, they would stop gaining weight.

The best way to lose weight, then, is to eat as you usually do—or less if your total calorie intake is excessive—only in smaller portions, broken up into small meals and snacks. Patients I put on diets are instructed to eat not only three meals a day, but three snacks as well.

Breakfast doesn't have to be large. Most of my patients aren't used to eating breakfast. Part of the problem comes from the fact that they are just not morning people, and part of it is that they are lazy. I tell them simply that they will have to set their alarms ten minutes earlier every day. Then they will have time to eat breakfast. Breakfast depends a lot on what you like. It can be a quick bowl of low-calorie cold cereal (puffed wheat or rice) and skim milk, or it can be Postum and one slice of bread with cheese.

The next assignment is a mid-morning snack. Half a grapefruit or a quarter of a cantaloupe will do fine. If that's not possible, take a wedge of cheese and a cracker or hard-boiled egg to work in your purse. You won't be so hungry for lunch then. Lunch should be a balance of protein and a vegetable or fruit, or both. Clear or vegetable soups are low in calories and are great fillers.

A late-afternoon snack is a must. First, it gives an energy pickup. Second, it comes at a time when not only are you beginning to drag, but your blood sugar is also beginning to sag. It prevents that mad dash to the refrigerator when you arrive home. It even gives you enough energy to plan a decent menu. This snack should occur at 3:30 or 4 P.M. Have some protein: yogurt, cottage cheese and melon, milk and a cracker, the other half of the can of tuna fish that you didn't finish for lunch, or a cup of soup. If you are a fruit lover, have an apple and take time for a cup of herbal tea. Slow down for a moment. Your body will thank you.

Again at dinner, eat lightly—some protein balanced by a vegetable and salad or fresh fruit. And don't omit a bedtime snack. A half-glass of skim milk is good, and it helps you sleep better.

If you are a working woman who has to make supper for your husband and your children, be smart. Take time and sit down for a moment and have your fruit cup (all fresh, of course) or your salad before you serve everyone else. As a mother and a provider, if your house works like many other houses, you are the one who always gets up during dinner to fetch this and that. My grandmother, who had eleven children, was an expert at eating first to fortify herself before dinner. Another possibility more appropriate to families in which both parents work outside the home is to have husband and children share the responsibility for food preparation and serving.

In any case, you should eat slowly and chew your food well. Serve it on salad plates so that the portions look bigger, and eat with smaller utensils—a salad fork or a demitasse spoon—so that you take smaller bites. Practice putting your fork down between bites, so that eating seems to take longer. Place a glass of water on the table and make sure that you finish it by the time your meal is over.

I never deny patients anything they like except heavy, gooey desserts, diet sodas and artificial sweeteners, and umpteen cups of coffee a day. Learn to drink water. Try it hot with the juice of a quarter of a lemon. Add a teaspoon of sugar; the eighteen calories will be used up by the time you stop stirring your hot lemonade. And learn to do without artificial sweeteners; enjoy the natural taste of food.

By the way, if you like oranges, you should be aware that although they are good for you, they contain many calories. One per day is enough. I have had several patients who dieted but drank several glasses of orange juice per day and wondered why they never lost weight. Substitute lower calorie juices such as grapefruit or tomato, or better yet, water.

Most women know what they should eat and what they shouldn't. My instructions are simply: eat what you like, eat less of it, and divide it up over three meals and three snacks.

Dieters always want to lose twenty pounds yesterday. Therefore, they get discouraged easily. They come in to the office after two weeks and lament that they have lost only four pounds. As far as I am concerned, that is perfect. I explain that losing two pounds per week would add up to a 104-pound weight loss in one year, and few of my patients have that much to lose. That simple calculation usually makes everyone feel better about their weekly weight loss and puts their particular weight loss goals into proper perspective.

All my patients accuse me of not eating much. The truth is that I probably eat more than any two of them put together, but I have a well-balanced diet and never miss a meal. I rarely miss snack times, either. As a result, I weigh exactly what I weighed twenty years ago. That's a problem too, because all the clothes that I have ever bought still fit, and they sit there in my closet with no excuse to throw them out.

Rest

When you feel sick—rest. Your body is telling you that it needs a little attention and tender loving care. Many of my patients say, "I've had a sore throat and cough for a week. Please give me some penicillin so I can keep on going to work and also get to school tomorrow."

I tell them that there are no magic pills. Usually what they need even more than a doctor is to go to bed and let their bodies recuperate. Unfortunately, we live in an age when everyone is in a rush. No one has the time to get sick. We most often get sick when we are burning both ends of the candle. I know. I have had a great deal of experience in getting sick, especially when I was in medical school. It has taught me that if I begin to drag or get a sore throat, I should take it easy and make sure that I get proper rest. I know what happens when I keep on pushing. I have had pneumonia twice and many years of catching whatever my patients walked in the door with, so I have gotten smarter in my old age, and now I listen to my body. I also caution my patients to avoid crowded places such as movie theaters when they are run-down or when the flu is epidemic.

I saw a new young patient not long ago. She had lost fourteen pounds and was having symptoms of colitis. She was attending college and holding down two jobs. One kept her up until 2 A.M. twice a week, the other job was just for experience. Finding nothing wrong physically, I sat her down for a long talk.

"Tell me," I said, "why must you carry a full-time schedule in school plus two part-time jobs?"

Her answer was simply, "I like doing all of these things."

"But you're ruining your health. As a matter of fact, if you continue, I guarantee that you will have colitis just like your brother. Now," I said, "what is the most important thing that you are doing?"

"College," she said.

"And the next?"

"Well, the evening job," and then she quickly added, "but I love the afternoon work, too. It's interesting."

After a few moments of conversation, we had determined that one job was definitely more satisfying than the other, and that it was sufficient for her economic needs.

She quit her other job the very next day. She has gained back ten pounds. She smiles and no longer looks haggard. Her "colitis" disappeared within two weeks.

It is important to know what is really vital. Some people never learn this and continue running in circles, faster and faster. They are constantly frustrated, exhausted, and never really accomplish anything important because they have spread themselves too thin. Know yourself, determine your goals, and stick to them.

IN CONCLUSION

All women are my sisters, and I want them to have the very best health care. The means of achieving good health care are in the hands of women themselves. The medical community has always been slow and reluctant to change. We must *force* change, so that medical care for women becomes more humane and less authoritarian.

I have written this book in the hope that it will give you the medical background you need to play an assertive role. I will consider my effort successful when women begin to question a diagnosis, its implications, and the appropriateness of the suggested therapy.

I feel that women in medicine have a special responsibility to educate women. Female physicians should speak out on medical and surgical practices that adversely affect other women. They should be in the forefront, making it possible for women to defend themselves against unnecessary hysterectomies or radical mastectomies. They should speak out against the medical mythology that discriminates against women—such as that menstrual pain is something that occurs because you don't like being female.

The sexist attitudes of the medical community all too often interfere with adequate care for women. Women can only improve their care when they know the facts and are able to participate intelligently in their own care. Women need information, not just a pat on the head or the back.

Impetus for change in the world of medicine in general and gynecology in particular can be generated by educating women to create pressure for better and more enlightened care. I have tried to hold up my end of this trust. Now it's your turn. With our combined efforts, we can succeed.

Notes

CHAPTER 1   NO MORE MENSTRUAL CRAMPS

1. A. Schwartz, U. Zor, H. R. Lindner, and S. Naor, "Primary Dysmenorrhea," *Journal of Obstetrics/Gynecology* 44, 5 (November 1974): 709–12.
2. V. R. Pickles, "Prostaglandins and Aspirin," *Nature* 239 (1972): 33–34.
3. Emil Novak and E. R. Novak, *Textbook of Gynecology* (Baltimore, Md.: Williams & Wilkins, 1952).
4. John I. Brewer, *Textbook of Gynecology* (Baltimore, Md.: Williams & Wilkins, 1961).
5. Langdon Parsons and Sheldon C. Sommers, *Gynecology*, 2nd ed. (Philadelphia: W. B. Saunders, 1978).
6. V. R. Pickles, W. J. Hall, F. A. Best, and G. N. Smith, "Prostaglandins in Endometrium and Menstrual Fluid from Normal and Dysmenorrheic Subjects," *British Journal of Obstetrics/Gynecology* 72 (1965): 185–92.
7. W. W. Fox, *Lancet* 1 (1953): 195.
8. G. G. Hill, Letter to the Editor, *British Medical Journal* (28 June 1975).
9. John R. Vane, "Inhibition of Prostaglandin Synthesis as a Mechanism of Action for Aspirin-like Drugs," *Nature* 231 (1971): 232–35.
10. Schwartz, Zor, Lindner, and Naor, "Primary Dysmenorrhea," 710–11.

11. Penny W. Budoff, "Unique Health Problems of Women in Industry," in *Women in Industry,* ed. Pasquale A. Carone, Sherman N. Kieffer, Leonard W. Krinsky, and Stanley F. Yolles (Albany: State University of New York Press, 1977): 154–67.

12. Penny W. Budoff, "Treatment of Dysmenorrhea," *American Journal of Obstetrics and Gynecology* 129 (15 September 1977): 232.

13. M. D. Chesney and D. L. Tasto, "The Development of the Menstrual Symptom Questionnaire," *Behavior, Research & Therapy* 13 (1975): 237–44.

14. Penny W. Budoff, "Use of Mefenamic Acid in the Treatment of Primary Dysmenorrhea," *Journal of the American Medical Association* 241, 25 (22 June 1979): 2713–16.

15. W. T. Beaver, T. G. Kanton, and G. Levy, "Putting Aspirin to Its Many Good Uses," *Patient Care* 13, 15 (15 September 1979): 70.

16. A. C. Turnbull, ed., *Research and Clinical Forums* 1, 2 (1979): 1–137.

17. Nils Wiquist, ed., *Acta Obstetricia et Gynecologica Scandinavica,* supplement 87 (1979): 1–117.

CHAPTER 2   NO MORE PREMENSTRUAL SYNDROME

1. Robert A. H. Kinch, "Help for Patients with Premenstrual Tension," *Consultant* (April 1979): 187–91.

2. M. L. Belfer and M. Carroll, *Archives of General Psychiatry* 25 (1971): 540.

3. Frank Seixas, "Spotting the Female Alcoholic," *Female Patient* (February 1976): 49–52.

4. Kinch, "Help for Patients with Premenstrual Tension."

5. Katharina Dalton, *Once a Month* (New York: Hunter House, 1979).

6. Gwyneth A. Sampson, "Premenstrual Syndrome: A Double-Blind Controlled Trial of Progesterone and Placebo," *British Journal of Psychiatry* 135 (1979): 209–15.

7. W. M. Herrmann and R. C. Beach, "Experimental and Clinical Data Indicating the Psychotropic Properties of Progestogens," *Postgraduate Medical Journal* 54, supplement 2 (1978): 82–87.

8. Ibid.

9. P. M. Leary and Kathleen Batho, "Changes in the Electroencephalogram Related to the Menstrual Cycle," *South African Medical Journal* 55 (21 April 1979): 666–68.

10. Personal communication with Sandoz Pharmaceuticals.
11. Bernard J. Carroll and Meir Steiner, "The Psychobiology of Premenstrual Dysphoria: The Role of Prolactins," *Psychoneuroendocrinology* 3 (1978): 174.
12. M. D. Baumblatt and F. Winston, "Pyridoxine and the Pill," *Lancet* 1 (1970): 833.
13. J. Stokes and J. Mendels, "Pyridoxine and Premenstrual Tension," *Lancet* 1 (1972): 1177–78.
14. Anthony H. Labrum, "Prolactin and Premenstrual Syndrome," *Female Patient* (July 1979): 76–84.
15. "Migraines and Prostaglandins," *Current Concepts in Pain and Analgesia* 5, 1: 4–11.
16. Bellergal, manufactured by Dorsey.
17. Penny W. Budoff, "Premenstrual Syndrome—Treatment with Mefenamic Acid," in press.
18. B. Andersch, L. Hahn, M. Anderson, and B. Isaksson, "Body Water and Weight in Patients with Premenstrual Tension," *British Medical Journal of Obstetrics and Gynaecology* 85 (July 1978): 546–50.
19. W. G. Wong et al., *American Journal of Obstetrics and Gynecology* 114 (1972): 950–53.
20. Sodium-restricted diet plan reprinted with permission from the Carnation Company, Los Angeles, Calif.
21. Andersch, Hahn, Anderson, and Isaksson, "Body Water and Weight."
22. Robert Bell, "Hormone Influences on Human Aggression," *Irish Journal of Medical Science* 147, supplement 1 (August 1978): 5–9.
23. Mary Louise Bunker and Margaret McWilliams, "Caffeine Content of Common Beverages," *Journal of the American Dietetic Association* 74 (January 1979): 28–32.
24. Ibid.
25. John P. Minton, M. K. Foecking, D. J. T. Webster, and R. H. Matthews, "Caffeine, Cyclic Nucleotides, and Breast Disease," *Surgery* 86, no. 1 (July 1979): 105–109.

CHAPTER 3   CONTRACEPTION: SAFE AT ANY AGE

1. Personal communication from I. Ronald Shenker, Associate Professor of Pediatrics at Long Island Jewish Hospital, New Hyde Park, N.Y.

2. Hershel Jick, M.D., et al., "Vaginal Spermicides and Congenital Disorders," *Journal of the American Medical Association* 245, 13: 1329–32.

3. Ibid.

4. Tatum-T intrauterine copper contraceptive package insert, Searle Laboratories, Chicago, Illinois.

5. *Population Council Reports of the Population Information Program of Johns Hopkins University,* vol. VII, series B, no. 3 (May 1979): 64.

6. Penny W. Budoff, Letter to the Editor, *Journal of the American Medical Association* (17 August 1979).

7. Jack Lippes, from speech given at Pre-FIGO Congress in Tokyo, Japan, October 1979: personal communication.

8. Tatum-T intrauterine copper contraceptive package insert, Searle Laboratories, Chicago, Illinois.

9. Irving Sivin, *Population Council Reports,* vol. VII, series B, no. 3 (May 1979): 71.

10. Christopher Tietze and Sarah Lewit, "Life Risks Associated with Reversible Methods of Fertility Regulation," *International Journal of Gynaecology and Obstetrics* 16.

11. "Oral Contraception," *Population Council Reports,* series A, no. 5 (January 1979).

12. Penny W. Budoff, "Unique Health Problems of Women in Industry," in *Women in Industry,* ed. Pasquale A. Carone, Sherman N. Kieffer, Leonard W. Krinsky, and Stanley F. Yolles (Albany: State University of New York Press, 1977): 154–67.

13. "Oral Contraception," *Population Council Reports,* series A, no. 5 (January 1979).

14. Usual oral contraceptive package inserts, FDA-approved precautions.

15. *Ob/Gyn News* (15 January 1980): 3.

16. *Sexual Medicine* (Washington, D.C.: International News Service, Inc., July 1978).

17. Robert A. Goepp, "Customized Cervical Caps." *Reports* (University of Chicago) 27, no. 2 (Spring 1979): 1–3.

18. Ibid.

CHAPTER 4   NO MORE RADICAL MASTECTOMIES

1. *Ob/Gyn News* (15 January 1980): 41.

2. *Journal of the American Medical Association* (6 July 1979): 14.

3. Dr. Frances Moore.

4. Langdon Parsons and Sheldon C. Sommers, *Gynecology*, 2nd ed. (Philadelphia: W. B. Saunders, 1978): 261.

5. Ibid., 1226.

6. Ibid., 1231.

7. C. H. Joseph Chang, *Emergency Medicine* (15 February 1980).

8. Minton, Foecking, Webster, and Matthews, "Caffeine, Cyclic Nucleotides, and Breast Disease."

9. Alan Bennett, "Prostaglandins in Relation to Human Endocrine and Breast Cancers," *Reviews on Endocrine-Related Cancer* 3 (1979): 5–10.

10. *The Breast Cancer Digest* (Bethesda, Md.: Office of Cancer Communications, National Cancer Institute, 1979): 29.

11. Budoff, "Unique Health Problems."

12. Marvin Rotman, Stephen Alderman, Madhu John, and Thomas Herskovic, "Radiation Therapy for Breast Cancer," *Journal of Reproductive Medicine* 23, no. 1 (July 1979): 13–20.

13. G. Bonadonna, U. Veronesi, and P. Valagusta, *Clinical Cancer Letter* 3, no. 10 (1980): 3.

14. A Szczeklik et al., "Prostacyclin in the Therapy of Peripheral Arterial Disease," in *Advances in Prostaglandin and Thromboxane Research* 7, ed. B. Samuelsson, P. Ramwell, and R. Paolette (New York: Raven Press, 1979): 687–89.

CHAPTER 5 NO MORE HOT FLASHES

1. Penny W. Budoff, "Unique Health Problems."

2. Herbert Kupperman, *Ob/Gyn News,* 15 November 1979.

3. Budoff, "Unique Health Problems," 154–67.

4. Ibid.

5. Dr. Sheldon C. Sommers.

6. Penny W. Budoff and Sheldon C. Sommers, "Estrogen-Progesterone Therapy in Perimenopausal Women," *Journal of Reproductive Medicine* 22, 5 (May 1979): 241–47.

7. Charles B. Hammond et al., "Effects of Long-Term Estrogen Replacement Therapy," *American Journal of Obstetrics and Gynecology* 133 (1979): 525.

8. R. K. Ross et al., "A Case-Control Study of Menopausal Estrogen Therapy and Breast Cancer," *Journal of the American Medical Association* 243, 16 (25 April 1980): 1635–39.

9. Paul Meier and Richard L. Landau, "Estrogen Replacement

Therapy," editorial in *Journal of the American Medical Association* 243, 16 (25 April 1980): 1658.

10. B. Hans Davidson, *Family Practice News* (15 October 1979): 36.

11. Meldrum, *Ob/Gyn News* (15 September 1979): 10.

12. P. L. Martin, S. S. C. Yen, A. M. Burnier, and H. Herrmann, "Systemic Absorption and Sustained Effects of Vaginal Estrogen Creams," *Journal of the American Medical Association* 242, 24 (14 December 1979): 2699–700.

13. Gilbert S. Gordon, *Ob/Gyn News* (1 July 1979): 16.

14. Lila E. Nachtigall, Richard H. Nachtigall, Robert D. Nachtigall, and E. Mark Beckman, "Estrogen Replacement Therapy," *Obstetrics and Gynecology 53*, 3 (March 1979): 277–80.

CHAPTER 6   KEEPING YOUR UTERUS AND KEEPING IT HEALTHY

1. Y. M. M. Bishop and F. Mosteller, "Smoothed Contingency Table Analysis," in *National Halothane Study*, ed. J. P. Bunker et al. (Bethesda, Md.: National Institutes of Health, 1969): 259–66.

2. John P. Bunker, Klim McPherson, and Philip L. Henneman, "Elective Surgery," in *Costs, Risks, and Benefits of Surgery*, ed. John P. Bunker (New York: Oxford University Press, 1977): 262–76.

3. Philip Cole and Joyce Berlin, "Elective Hysterectomy," *American Journal of Obstetrics and Gynecology* 129, 2 (15 September 1977): 117–23.

4. Ibid.

5. Ibid.

6. Irak M. Rutkow and George D. Zuidema, "Unnecessary Surgery," *Surgery* 84, 5 (November 1978): 671–77.

7. Frederick J. Hofmeister, "Ten Year Review of Hysterectomies," *American Journal of Obstectrics and Gynecology* 134, 4 (15 June 1979): 435.

8. Ibid.

9. Hassan Amirikia and T. N. Evans, "Ten Year Review of Hysterectomies: Trends, Indications, and Risks," *American Journal of Obstetrics and Gynecology* 134, 4 (15 June 1979): 431–34.

10. Ibid.

11. Penny W. Budoff, "A Progesterone IUD for Menorrhagia," *Female Patient* (May 1978): 79.
12. Langdon Parsons and Sheldon C. Sommers, *Gynecology*, 2nd ed. (Philadelphia: W. B. Saunders, 1978): 1281.
13. Ibid., 1051.
14. S. B. Gusberg and A. L. Kaplan, "Precursors of Corpus Cancer," *American Journal of Obstetrics and Gynecology* 87 (1963): 662.
15. Sheldon C. Sommers, "Pre-Malignant Lesions of the Endometrium," *The Practice of Surgery Series,* ed. Hugh R. K. Barber (New York: Harper & Row, in press).
16. Ibid.
17. Ibid.
18. Ibid.
19. B. Hark and Sheldon C. Sommers, "Endometrial Curettage in Diagnosis and Therapy," *Obstetrics and Gynecology* 21 (1963): 636.
20. Sommers, "Pre-Malignant Lesions."
21. Ibid.
22. Ibid.
23. Martha N. Gizynski, "Psychic Trauma of Gynecologic Surgery," *Female Patient* (February 1978): 37–39.
24. John E. Wennberg, "Factors Governing Utilization of Hospital Services," *Hospital Practice* 14, 9 (September 1979): 115–27.

CHAPTER 7   YOUR GYNECOLOGICAL EXAMINATION

1. Albert Singer and Bevan Reid, "Does the Male Transmit Cervical Cancer?" *Contemporary Ob/Gyn* 13 (April 1979): 173–80.
2. L. Martinez, "Relationship of Squamous Cell Carcinoma of the Cervic Uteri to Squamous Cell Carcinoma of the Penis," *Cancer* 24 (1969): 277.
3. I. Kessler, "Human Cervical Cancer as a Venereal Disease," *Cancer Research* 25 (1976): 783.
4. Singer and Reid, "Does the Male Transmit Cervical Cancer."
5. Roland A. Pattillo, A. C. F. Ruckert, M. T. Story, and R. F. Mattingly, "Immunodiagnosis in Ovarian Cancer: Blocking Factor Activity," *American Journal of Obstetrics and Gynecology* 133, 7 (1 April 1979).
6. Ross S. Berkowitz and Robert C. Knapp, "Early Detection of Ovarian Cancer," *Female Patient* (July 1979): 92–97.

7. Ibid.

8. Ibid.

9. James H. Gilbaugh, Jr., and Peter C. Fuchs, "The Gonococcus and the Toilet Seat," *New England Journal of Medicine* 301, 2 (12 July 1979): 91–93.

10. Paul J. Welcher, *Modern Medicine* (August 15–September 15, 1979): 87.

CHAPTER 8   BODY HOUSEKEEPING

1. R. Glynn, "Vaginal pH and the Effect of Douching," *Obstetrics and Gynecology* 23 (September 1962): 369–72.

2. Kathryn N. Shands et al., "Toxic Shock Syndrome in Menstruating Women: Its Association with Tampon Use and *Staphylococcus aureus* and the Clinical Features in 52 Cases," *New England Journal of Medicine* 303, 25 (18 December 1980): 1436–42.

3. Ibid.

Index